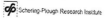

Progress in Inflammation Research

Series Editor

Prof. Dr. Michael J. Parnham
PLIVA
Research Institute
Prilaz baruna Filipovica 25
10000 Zagreb
Croatia

Forthcoming titles:
Anti-Inflammatory or Anti-Rheumatic Drugs, R.O. Day, D.E. Furst, P.L. Van Riel (Editors), 2003
Inflammatory Processes and Cancer, D.W. Morgan, U. Forssmann, M. Nakada (Editors), 2003
Inflammation and Cardiac Diseases, G.Z. Feuerstein (Editor), 2003

(Already published titles see last page.)

The Hereditary Basis of Allergic Diseases

Stephen T. Holgate
John W. Holloway

Editors

Birkhäuser Verlag
Basel · Boston · Berlin

Editors

Stephen T. Holgate
University of Southampton
School of Medicine
IIR (Respiratory Cell and Molecular Biology) Division
Southampton General Hospital
Southampton SO16 6YD
UK

John W. Holloway
University of Southampton
School of Medicine
Human Genetics and IIR (Respiratory Cell and Molecular Biology) Divisions
Southampton General Hospital
Southampton SO16 6YD
UK

A CIP catalogue record for this book is available from the Library of Congress, Washington D.C., USA

Deutsche Bibliothek Cataloging-in-Publication Data
The hereditary basis of allergic diseases / S. Holgate ; J. Holloway, ed.. -
Basel ; Boston ; Berlin : Birkhäuser, 2002
    (Progress in inflammation research)
    ISBN 3-7643-6402-5

The publisher and editor can give no guarantee for the information on drug dosage and administration contained in this publication. The respective user must check its accuracy by consulting other sources of reference in each individual case.

The use of registered names, trademarks etc. in this publication, even if not identified as such, does not imply that they are exempt from the relevant protective laws and regulations or free for general use.

ISBN 3-7643-6402-5 Birkhäuser Verlag, Basel – Boston – Berlin

© 2002 Birkhäuser Verlag, P.O. Box 133, CH-4010 Basel, Switzerland
Member of the BertelsmannSpringer Publishing Group
Printed on acid-free paper produced from chlorine-free pulp. TCF ∞
Cover design: Markus Etterich, Basel
Cover illustration: Typing of the interleukin-4 receptor alpha chain Q576R polymorphism using allele specific PCR reactions resolved on a 192-well ARMS-MADGE gel. Photo contributed by Dr. John W. Holloway.
Printed in Germany
ISBN 3-7643-6402-5

9 8 7 6 5 4 3 2 1

Contents

List of contributors

Lucien A. Aarden, Department of Auto-Immune Diseases, CLB and Laboratory for Experimental and Clinical Immunology, Academic Medical Center, University of Amsterdam, Plesmanlaan 125, 1066 CX Amsterdam, The Netherlands; e-mail: L_aarden@clb.nl

Chaker N. Adra, Beth Israel Deaconess Medical Center and The Children's Hospital, Harvard Medical School, Departments of Medicine and Pathology, Hematology/Oncology Division, 99 Brookline Avenue, Boston, MA 02215, USA; e-mail: cadra@caregroup.harvard.edu

Jeffrey M. Drazen, Division of Pulmonary and Critical Care Medicine, Brigham and Women's Hospital, 75 Francis Street, Boston, MA 02115, USA; e-mail: jdrazen@nejm.org

P.S. Gao, Experimental Medicine Unit, University of Wales Swansea, Swansea, UK; e-mail: gpsoy@yahoo.com

Hartmut Grasemann, Children's Hospital, University of Essen, Hufelandstrasse 55, 45122 Essen, Germany; e-mail: hartmutg@hotmail.com

Luigi Grasso, Morphotek Inc., 3624 Market Street, Philadelphia, PA 19104, USA; e-mail: grasso@morphotek.com

Nobuyuki Hizawa, First Department of Medicine, School of Medicine, Hokkaido University, Kita-Ku, N-15 W-7, Sapporo 060-8638, Japan; e-mail: nhizawa@med.hokudai.ac.jp

John W. Holloway, University of Southampton, School of Medicine, Human Genetics and IIR (Respiratory Cell and Molecular Biology) Divisions, Southampton General Hospital, Southampton SO16 6YD, UK; e-mail: j.w.holloway@soton.ac.uk

J.M. Hopkin, Experimental Medicine Unit, University of Wales Swansea, Swansea, UK; e-mail: J.M.Hopkin@Swansea.ac.uk

Ladina Joos, UBC Pulmonary Research Laboratory, St. Paul's Hospital, 1081 Burrard Street, Vancouver, B.C., Canada, V6Z 1Y6

Tarja Laitinen, Department of Medical Genetics, University of Helsinki, Haartmaninkatu 8 (Box 63), 00014 Helsinki, Finland; e-mail: tarja.laitinen@helsinki.fi

Roy C. Levitt, Genaera Institute of Molecular Medicine, Genaera Corporation, 5110 Campus Drive, Plymouth Meeting, PA 19462, USA; e-mail: rlevitt@genaera.com

Adel H. Mansur, Molecular Medicine Unit, Clinical Sciences Building, St. James's University Hospital, Leeds LS9 7TF, UK; e-mail: adelmansur@hotmail.com

X.-Q. Mao, Department of Health Promotion and Human Behaviour, Kyoto University Graduate School of Public Health, Kyoto, Japan; and Experimental Medicine Unit, University of Swansea, Swansea, UK; e-mail: xqmao@swansea.ac.uk

Michael P. McLane, Genaera Institute of Molecular Medicine, Genaera Corporation, 5110 Campus Drive, Plymouth Meeting, PA 19462, USA; e-mail: MMcLane@Genaera.com

Nicholas C. Nicolaides, Morphotek Inc., 3624 Market Street, Philadelphia, PA 19104, USA; e-mail: nicolaides@morphotek.com

Carole Ober, Department of Human Genetics, The University of Chicago, 920 East 58th Street, Room 507C, Chicago, IL 60627, USA; e-mail: c-ober@genetics.uchicago.edu

Peter D. Paré, UBC Pulmonary Research Laboratory, St. Paul's Hospital, 1081 Burrard Street, Vancouver, B.C., Canada, V6Z 1Y6; e-mail: ppare@mrl.ubc.ca

A.P. Sampson, Respiratory Cell and Molecular Biology Research Division, Southampton General Hospital, Tremona Road, Southampton, SO16 6YD, UK; e-mail: aps@soton.ac.uk

Andrew J. Sandford, UBC Pulmonary Research Laboratory, St. Paul's Hospital, 1081 Burrard Street, Vancouver, B.C., Canada, V6Z 1Y6; e-mail: asandford@mrl.ubc.ca

Ian Sayers, Human Genetics Research Division, Southampton General Hospital, Tremona Road, Southampton, SO16 6YD, UK;
e-mail: Dr_Ian_Sayers@hotmail.com

Taro Shirakawa, Department of Health Promotion and Human Behaviour, Kyoto University Graduate School of Public Health, Kyoto, Japan; and Experimental Medicine Unit, University of Swansea, Swansea, UK;
e-mail: shirakawa@pbh.med.kyoto-u.ac.jp

Tineke C.T.M. van der Pouw Kraan, Department of Molecular Cell Biology, Faculty of Medicine, Free University Amsterdam, Van der Boechorststraat 7, 1081 BT Amsterdam, The Netherlands; e-mail: T.van_der_pouw_kraan.cell@med.vu.nl

Jaring S. van der Zee, Department of Pulmology, F3N Academic Medical Center, University of Amsterdam, Meibergdreef 9, 1105 AZ Amsterdam, The Netherlands; e-mail: J.S.vanderZee@Amc.uva.nl

Matthias Wjst, Gruppe Molekulare Epidemiologie, Institut für Epidemiologie, GSF – Forschungszentrum für Umwelt und Gesundheit, Ingolstädter Landstrasse 1, D-85758 Neuherberg/Munich, Germany; e-mail: m@wjst.de

Akiko Yamasaki, Department of Health Promotion and Human Behaviour, Kyoto University Graduate School of Public Health, Kyoto, Japan;
e-mail: otsu-tky@umin.ac.jp

Xing Yang, Beth Israel Deaconess Medical Center, Harvard Medical School, Hematology/Oncology Division, 99 Brookline Avenue, Boston, MA 02215, USA; e-mail: xyang@caregroup.harvard.edu

Preface

Allergic diseases are complex and involve a range of environmental factors interacting with a susceptible genotype. The familial clustering of diseases, such as asthma and hay fever, have been recognised for over two centuries, but the basis for this has had to await the molecular biological revolution. Estimates of the contribution that genetic factors make to asthma susceptibility range from 35–70%. For the majority of allergic diseases, segregation analysis has not identified a consistent Mendelian pattern of inheritance, which, when combined with multiple phenotypes and environmental interactions, has made identifying candidate genes especially difficult and, at times, controversial. Part of the difficulty has been lack of agreement over phenotype definitions, reduced power of studies to predict linkage and association, and, importantly, lack of true heterogeneity between populations.

Despite these difficulties, the last decade has witnessed enormous progress in this field. *The Hereditary Basis of Allergic Diseases* brings together scholarly reviews of the emergent and promising genetic factors influencing susceptibility to and progression of allergic diseases such as asthma. There are important, up-to-date contributions on the understanding of the heritable basis of atopy and asthma phenotypes (Tarja Laitinen), and these have been used to undertake genome-wide searches to identify linkage to specific chromosomal regions (Mathias Wjst). The importance of immune regulatory responses is highlighted by focused contributions on genetic regulation of specific immunoglobulin E (IgE) responses and the importance of human leucocyte antigen (HLA) and T-cell receptor variation and altered signalling through FcεR1 receptors.

The recognition that allergic disorders result from an imbalance between Th1 and Th2 cytokines in favour of the latter provides the basis for further key chapters. This includes chapters on interleukin (IL)-13 polymorphism (Tineke Van der Pouw-Kraan and colleagues) and a contribution from Roy Levitt and colleagues on the role of polymorphism in the IL-9/IL-9R system in asthma. The target tissue in which an allergic disease expresses itself is also subject to genetic influences. Thus, genetic factors influencing asthma severity and bronchial hyper-responsiveness are well covered by Peter Paré and colleagues.

It is not possible to refer to allergic disease without considering the role of individual mediators. The leukotriene pathway is especially relevant to asthma, and the recent identification of polymorphism in some of the synthetic enzymes has not only helped sub-phenotype asthma, e.g., aspirin-intolerant asthma and the A–444C polymorphism of the LTC_4 synthase promoter, but, as pointed out by Ian Sayers and Tony Sampson, also provides a basis for drug variation in therapeutic responses. A mediator that has attracted much recent interest in asthma and rhinitis is nitric oxide. The recent identification of genetic variants in the nitric oxide synthase enzymes, as described by Drs Grasemann and Drazen, is of considerable interest.

The ongoing research into genetic factors behind the development and pathogenesis of atopy and allergic disease, as exemplified by the studies described in this book, will in due course provide us with a greater understanding of the fundamental mechanisms of these disorders. Study of these genetic factors in large longitudinal cohorts with extensive environmental information will allow the identification of both the environmental factors that in susceptible individuals trigger allergic disease and the periods of life in which this occurs, potentially leading to prevention of disease by environmental modification. Identification of genetic variants that predispose to allergic disease will result in several outcomes. First, the greater understanding of the susceptibility factors for the disease will allow development of specific new drugs both to relieve and prevent symptoms. In addition, different genetic variants may also influence the response to therapy. The identification of individuals with altered response to current drug therapies will allow optimisation of current therapeutic measures. Second, the identification of susceptibility factors for allergic disease will allow early identification of susceptible individuals, thus allowing them to be targeted at an early age for both therapy and environmental intervention such as avoidance of allergen exposure. Thus, genetic screening in early life may become a practical and cost-effective option in preventing allergic disease.

Overall, this book provides a comprehensive approach to advancing the understanding of the genetic factors influencing allergy. With the unravelling of the code of the human genome, the identification of the 27,000 or so genes, of which almost 60% are still with unknown function, will provide an ample challenge for the future. As scientists embark on further mining this extraordinary set of data, it is rewarding that already good progress is being made in uncovering genes involved in a disease area that touches almost everyone at some time in their lives. We are extremely grateful for all the time and effort that the authors have put into their chapters, which, as a consequence, led to a state-of-the-art publication in this field.

Stephen T. Holgate
John W. Holloway

Heredity of allergy and asthma

Tarja Laitinen

Department of Medical Genetics, University of Helsinki, Haartmaninkatu 8 (Box 63), 00014 Helsinki, Finland

Twin and family studies

Genetic vs environmental components in atopic disorders

Multiple population-based family and twin studies have shown genetic predisposition in asthma and other atopic disorders, although the mode of inheritance and contributing genes are unknown. It is likely that the set of contributing genes, the mode of inheritance, and the significance of genes compared to environmental factors differ between the patient groups. In other words, in these diseases, the molecular-genetic background is more complex than the diagnostic characteristics created for clinical purposes. In multifactorial diseases, the significance of genetic factors is often measured by sibling risk (λ_{sib}). Sibling risk is defined as the risk of a co-sibling becoming affected, if his or her sibling is already affected, divided by the risk of the population at large. For asthma, the λ_{sib} values vary depending on the characteristics of the study population. In Australia, $\lambda_{sib} = 3.5$ has been reported among adult siblings, while among 16-year-old dizygotic twins in Finland, λ_{sib} value was as high as 5 [1, 2]. Those two estimates show still a rather weak genetic effect compared with λ_{sib} values reported in other multifactorial diseases such as $\lambda_{sib} = 15$ in diabetes type I, $\lambda_{sib} = 60$ in celiac disease, or $\lambda_{sib} = 20$ in multiple sclerosis [3].

Asthma, however, is more frequent than the above-mentioned disorders, and using λ_{sib} values as the only measure can underestimate the significance of genetic factors in the development of asthma. λ_{sib} values are forced to decrease when a disease becomes more common in the population. For example, for the prevalences 1%, 5%, and 10%, the corresponding λ_{sib} values that cannot be exceeded are 100, 20, and 10, respectively. On the other hand, familial aggregation of asthma does not necessarily imply genetic transmission; shared environmental factors might also be of importance. These components can be distinguished by comparing pair-wise concordance rates of genetically identical monozygotic (MZ) and dizygotic (DZ) twins who represent full sibs (or other groups of pairs that share the same environment but differ genetically). If all MZ twins (sibs that share the whole genome) and 50% of DZ twins (sibs that share on average half of the genome) are concordant, a dis-

The Hereditary Basis of Allergic Diseases, edited by Stephen T. Holgate and John W. Holloway
© 2002 Birkhäuser Verlag Basel/Switzerland

ease is fully genetically regulated (heritability 100%). In common diseases such as asthma, the heritability is reduced when one estimates the proportion of genetic factors compared with shared and individual environmental factors in the development of the disease.

For asthma there is an interesting and comparable series of studies recently done in Nordic countries (Tab. 1) [2, 4–6]. They are all nation-wide questionnaire-based studies with high response rates done among young-age cohorts; in all countries, the questionnaires included a broad spectrum of questions on health and lifestyle. Therefore, it is unlikely that the surveys are biased by better response rates from atopic families. All studies show a high (62–79%) genetic component in the development of asthma. In fact, the genetic component was higher than in Nordic studies done before the rapid increase of atopic disorders in industrialized countries (44–63%) [7, 8]. At the time of the first Finnish study among adult twin pairs (at the age of 28 to 80, born before year 1958, and both twins alive in 1967), the prevalence of asthma was 1.6% and the genetic effect was 44% in the development of asthma. In the latter study, the twins were born from 1975 to 1979 and were studied at the age of 16. The prevalence of asthma was 3.9% and the proportion of genetic factors was estimated higher (65–79%) in the liability of asthma. The higher heredity can be explained by a higher uniformity in environmental exposures compared with previous studies done among adults or by early onset of the disease predicting higher genetic susceptibility among adolescents than among mixed age groups. Most importantly, however, the increase of asthma has not decreased the importance of genetic factors. Aggregation of asthma into families is still caused mainly because of genetic rather than shared environmental factors. Twin studies have shown a significant genetic component also in the development of atopic exema and hay fever [9, 10].

Mode of inheritance in atopic disorders

The mode of inheritance can be studied only in family settings by means of segregation analysis [11]. Segregation analysis is used to analyze the pattern of inheritance of a disorder by observing how the disease is distributed within families. The number of affected individuals is compared with the expected number using different analytical models of inheritance. Confounding factors, such as selecting models of inheritance that explain poorly true inheritance of the disease and errors in phenotyping, decrease the power of the analysis. Because of uncertainties in phenotyping, especially when digotomized clinical phenotypes are used, several research groups have chosen to study segregation of asthma-associated quantitative traits. Those studies have shown that many of these traits are under genetic control and that many of the models favor major loci (Mendelian components) in autosomes acting against polygenic background [11]. Using variance components analysis, high

Table 1 - Recent Nordic population-based twin studies showing relatively high genetic component in the development of asthma

Country	Year of study	Number of twin pairs	Individual response rate	Age (years) of twins	Definition of asthma in the questionnaire	Prevalence of asthma in the study populations	Heritability of asthma
Norway	1992	2,570	73%	18–25	Ever asthma	6%[1] and 5%[2]	75%
Sweden	1994	1,339	90%[3]	7–9	Ever or current asthma	18%[1] and 10%[2]	76%[1] and 62%[2]
Finland	1991–94	1,713	81%	16	Diagnosed by a physician	4%	79%
Denmark	1994	12,352	86%	12–41	Ever asthma	6%	73%

[1]among males; [2]among females; [3]questionnaires were sent to the parents

heritability has been reported for both high serum total IgE (47%) and specific serum IgE levels against timothy and house dust mite (34%), for blood eosinophil counts (30%), and for bronchial hyperreactivity (30%) [12, 13]. Even though these traits occur highly correlated among patients suffering allergic symptoms, it is unclear to what extent these traits are under the same genetic control. Interestingly, the comparison of 23 genome scans done in different autoimmune/immune diseases including asthma showed that the positive linkages map non-randomly into 18 distinct loci, suggesting that a common set of susceptibility genes may control the development of different immune diseases [14]. Therefore, it is possible that immune disorders with different target organs are genetically more related than, e.g., increased bronchial hyperreactivity and serum IgE level that have been suggested to be inherited independently [12]. Therefore, the primary recruitment criteria of the study families might be of great importance when the inheritance of atopy-associated phenotypes are analyzed.

In the Finnish twin families, the risk of asthma and hay fever was almost the same in parent-offspring pairs (3- to 4-fold risk) as it was in sibling-pairs (4- to 5-fold risk), favoring a dominant rather than recessive mode of inheritance [2, 10]. When we divided the 16-year-old twins into two different groups according to their parents' asthma status and repeated the twin modeling, the effect of genetic factors in asthma increased to 87% in the group of twins with an affected parent. In the group of twins with un-affected parents, the heritability was 52–76% [2]. Moreover, in the latter group, the model that accounted for only environmental factors explained the results as well, suggesting complexity among the families in the mode of inheritance of asthma.

Mendelian principles in complex traits

Atopic disorders or their quantitative phenotypes are not inherited in Mendelian fashion, but, in order to to focus our thinking, the studied phenotype can be considered a sum effect of different loci – predisposing or protective – that behave according to the same principals found in monogenic diseases (Fig. 1). However, the mode of recessive or dominant inheritance and penetrance of susceptibility alleles can vary between the loci. Furthermore, in one gene, several different susceptibility alleles may exist. Those alleles may also differ in their mode of inheritance and cause differences in the clinical picture of the disease. For example, congenital hyperinsulinism (OMIM #256450) is caused by mutations in the sulfonylurea receptor type 1. All reported mutations have been inherited recessively except for a missense mutation, E1506K, that is found to be heterozygous among the patients and causes a mild, but highly penetrant, form of the disease [15].

The contributing loci most likely affect in the development of the disease with varying influences. By being key molecules in the pathogenesis of a disease, some

Dominant	Recessive
Already one susceptibility allele in either parental chromosome increases the risk of asthma.	A susceptibility allele is needed in both maternal and paternal chromosomes before the risk of asthma is increased.

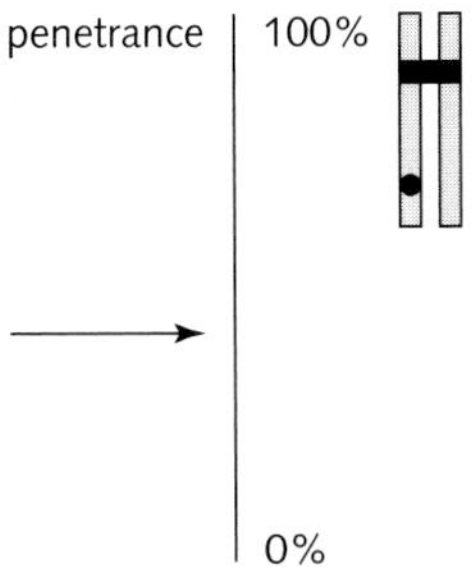

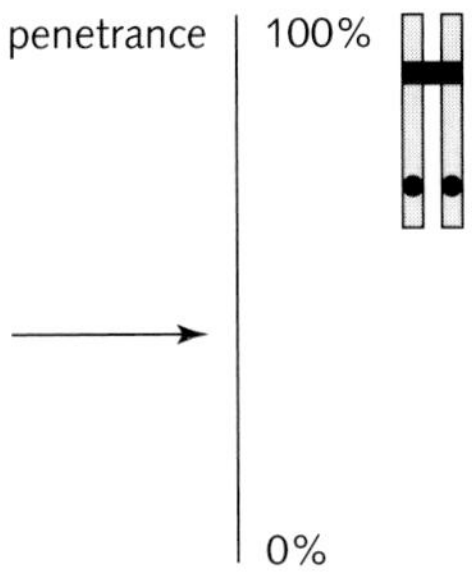

penetrance | 100%

penetrance | 100%

0%

0%

| If the gene acts in dominant fashion with 50% reduced penetrance, it means that still 50% of the individuals who carry the susceptibility allele are asymptomatic. | If the gene acts in recessive fashion with 50% reduced penetrance, it means that all the individuals who carry only one copy of the susceptibility allele are asymptomatic and 50% of the individuals who have the susceptibility allele in their both chromosomes are asymptomatic. |

- In polygonic diseases the phenotype is a sum effect of multiple susceptibility and – possibly also – protective loci that all act in Mendelian fashion but can have different patterns of inheritance or penetrance.
- The specific mechanisms for reduced penetrance in most of diseases are unknown, but gene-gene and gene-environment interactions are considered important.
- Based on family studies the risk of asthma in the proband is an affected parent and an affected sibling increase equally, the inheritance of asthma might be better explained by dominant than by recessive loci.

Figure 1
Although polygenetic disorders such as asthma do not follow the Mendelian patterns of inheritance, the genetic effect of each disease-associated locus in polygenetic disease follows the dominant or recessive pattern of inheritance with varying penetrance. The patterns of inheritance can differ among the contributing loci.

loci can notably increase the risk of the disease on their own (major loci), while some of the loci (minor loci) can become of significance only together with major genetic determinants or in extremely unfavorable environmental conditions. However, the weak regulators can become of great importance in certain combinations and increase the risk of the disease more than additively expected (epistasis in the gene-gene interactions). It has also been proposed that maternally inherited suspectibility allele can increase the risk of atopic disorders more than those inherited from the father by genetic mechanisms, such as imprinting, or by maternal modification of the developing infant's immune system [12].

Reduced penetrance and susceptibility alleles in complex traits

In most of the multifactorial disorders, the specific mechanisms of penetrance, interactions between susceptibility alleles, and interactions between genes and environmental factors are not known. In addition to epistasis, remarkably reduced penetrance compared with that found in monogenic traits has been proposed to be one of the main characteristics in the inheritance of polygenic traits. Familial primary pulmonary hypertension is caused by mutations in the BMPR2 gene (OMIM#178600). Lately, germline mutations in the same gene have been described among sporadic cases also [16]. These observations make the interface between hereditary and sporadic cases in primary pulmonary hypertension vague and show evidence of remarkably reduced penetrance of the identified mutations. Reduced penetrance in atopic disorders is supported by our own observation among the MZ twins. Only 8 of 30 MZ pairs were concordant for asthma, and 41 of 95 MZ pairs were concordant for allergic rhinitis, which is equivalent to penetrances of 27% for asthma and 43% for allergic rhinitis, respectively [2, 10]. These results, of course, do not give us direct information of penetrance of a solitary locus, which can be highly variable.

The difference between the terms "disease-causing mutation" and "susceptibility allele" is sometimes difficult to determine. If a genetic defect destroys the gene structure and, as a result, no stabile protein is translated and the disease phenotype is developed regardless of how favorable the environmental conditions are, it can be called a true disease-causing mutation based on both structural and functional grounds. These kinds of genetic defects are extremely rare in the population and most likely do not explain common diseases. Single nucleotide substitutions known to be very common [17, 18] in the human genome usually save the gene structure but cause changes in the affinity or activity of the protein or a decrease in expression level either by reduced production or reduced stability of the protein. These genetic defects are usually called DNA-level susceptibility alleles, and they increase the risk of diseases through altered function or expression of the protein. Obviously, an alternative or parallel signaling pathway in a favorable environment can sometimes substitute these defects. Based on these assumptions, it is easier to understand the remarkably reduced penetrance in complex traits and how the contributing genes are linked to environmental changes.

Simplified disease modeling

Because a deeper understanding of segregation analyses requires a lot of background knowledge of the method, a very simple model of inheritance of asthma is presented here to clarify how genetic effects of different loci may act. As a starting point for our asthma model, we can use the parameters from the Finnish twin study: the prevalence of 4% that can also be considered the risk of asthma at the age of 16 in

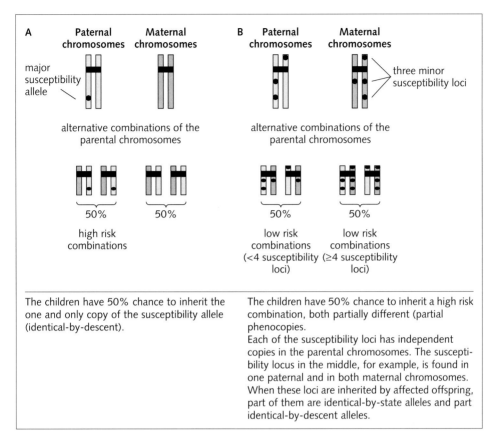

Figure 2
Two simplified models of the inheritance of asthma, in which there is (A) only one major locus or (B) multiple minor loci contributing to the development of the disease.

Finland and the sibling risk of 5-fold, which means the prevalence (or risk) of 20% among the siblings of the proband. Actually, the increased sibling risk can be explained easily with one dominant locus with 55% reduced penetrance (Fig. 2A). A genome-wide screen for asthma genes combined with linkage analysis should be efficient tools to identify these loci, but the results of the published studies so far show contrary evidence: several loci have been reported, the reported loci differ between ethnic groups, and the strength of linkage to all loci has remained rather low [19–24]. These results suggest that, at population level, tens of different loci are involved in the development of asthma and that significant locus heterogeneity exists between the study families. If major loci are involved in the development of asthma, contributing genes differ between the families and the genetic effect of distinct loci is diluted when data from different families are pooled.

Keeping in mind the prevalence of asthma and the hypothesis of several distinct major susceptibility loci, the frequency of each susceptibility locus has to be low in the population-based controls (< 1%) (Fig. 3). Therefore, it is unlikely that in the pool of parental chromosomes there is more than one copy of the allele (e.g., if the allele frequency is 1%, the likelihood for two copies is 0.01%). This restricts the possibilities to explain the observed sibling risk by several equally important loci. The offspring have a 25% chance to inherit two non-linked, identical-by-descent (IBD) alleles simultaneously and both alleles have to be fully penetrant to fill in the model. The likelihood of inheriting three IBD alleles simultaneously is 12.5%, and it does not explain the observed sibling risk.

If multiple equally important loci are needed in the development of asthma, the susceptibility alleles have to be common in the population, and copies of alleles (identical-by-state (IBS) alleles) can be found in the pool of parental chromosomes (Fig. 2B). Then an offspring has again a chance of 50% to inherit a combination of parental chromosomes with high number of susceptibility alleles. However, if susceptibility alleles are frequent in normal population (> 5%), their distinct genetic effect in the development of the disease has to be minor (Fig. 3). That also means that the pattern of susceptibility alleles may differ between an affected sib pair. Rare minor alleles may exist, but alone they do not explain the observed sibling risk in asthma. Extremely large genetic studies are needed before those loci can be identified, and, from a genetic point of view, they are of less importance.

Strategies in genetic studies

Based on family studies, both oligogenic and multigenic models at the patient or family level are equally probable, and, most importantly, they do not exclude one another (Fig. 4). It is possible that there is one major locus in the family and additional minor loci that modify the clinical picture of the disease. Even though it can be argued that both of these models are overly simplified and do not take into account many genetic phenomena of inheritance, understanding of these hypotheses can be helpful when genetic studies are designed and results are analyzed.

Assuming that at the patient level asthma is caused by one or few major loci, the susceptibility alleles have to be rather rare in the population; most likely, the affected pedigree members share an IBD locus. If we then are able to minimize locus heterogeneity among the study families, gene mapping and linkage analysis can be considered state-of-the-art-methods to identify the contributing genes. In this model, differences in the clinical outcome of the disease within a family are explained by environmental factors and individual genetic makeup (minor loci). Observations in monogenic diseases allow us to make this assumption. For example, neurofibro-

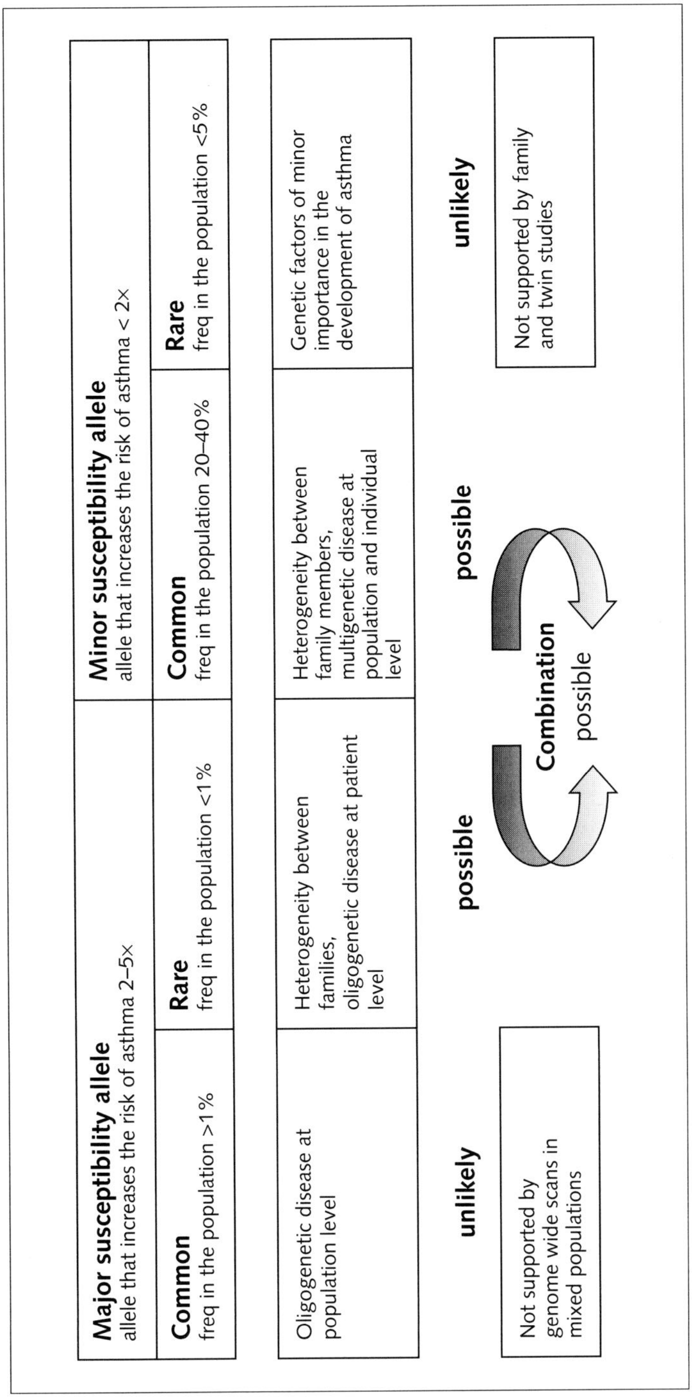

	Major susceptibility allele allele that increases the risk of asthma 2–5×		**Minor susceptibility allele** allele that increases the risk of asthma < 2×	
	Common freq in the population >1%	**Rare** freq in the population <1%	**Common** freq in the population 20–40%	**Rare** freq in the population <5%
	Oligogenetic disease at population level	Heterogeneity between families, oligogenetic disease at patient level	Heterogeneity between family members, multigenetic disease at population and individual level	Genetic factors of minor importance in the development of asthma
	unlikely	possible	possible	unlikely
	Not supported by genome wide scans in mixed populations			Not supported by family and twin studies

Combination possible

Figure 3
Oligogenic and multigenic model of the inheritance of asthma.

9

Oligogenic model of inheritance	Multigenic model of inheritance
several susceptibility loci at population level	
• In the population susceptibility alleles are rare (< 1%), but each of the alleles increases the the risk of disease 2–5 × compared to the risk in population at large (major susceptibility alleles).	• In the population susceptibility alleles are common (20–40%), but none of the alleles will increase the risk of a disease more than 2× compared to the risk in the population at large (minor susceptibility alleles).
• In each family, there is usually only one susceptibility allele (locus homogeneity between the family members).	• To become affected many susceptibility alleles of different loci have to be inherited at the same time (locus heterogeneity between the family members).
• If the genetic heterogeneity between families could be identified, mapping of susceptibility genes can be done efficiently using linkage analysis.	• Increased sibling risk can be explained by multiple susceptibility alleles inherited from either of the parents simultaneously.

• Attempts to solve genetic heterogeneity between the study families:
- by patient selection:
   narrowed phenotypes
   subphenotypes
   asthma associated quantitative traits
   early onset of the disease
   several family members affected
- by population selection:
   founder populations
	• The alleles are difficult to be identified by using linkage analysis, since siblings can be affected due to separate profiles of susceptibility alleles (partial phenocopies).
	
	• Large association studies are needed for the detection of the alleles and those studies demand prior knowledge on
	- relevant signalling pathways in the development of asthma
	- polymorphic structures of the signalling genes and their functional significance

Figure 4
Rough estimates for the frequencies of major and minor susceptibility alleles in the popula-
tion and probabilities of different models of inheritance in asthma.

matosis (OMIM#162200), which is caused by autosomal dominant mutations in the NF1 gene, has variable expression within an affected sibpair carrying the same mutation and sharing a lot of environmental factors. Expression may vary even more between different mutations, and, in the extreme ends, different mutations are known to cause totally different clinical phenotypes [25–27].

If we assume that asthma is caused by multiple loci acting simultaneously, susceptibility alleles have to be common in the population-based controls as well. Therefore, it is unlikely that all the affected family members have inherited an identical pattern of susceptibility alleles; the differences in the clinical picture are found as a result of true phenocopies of the disease. Even if similar susceptibility alleles are inherited by an affected sib pair, the alleles are not necessarily IBD (the same copy of the allele) but rather IBS (a similar but different copy of the allele). Phenocopies, especially if combined with reduced penetrance, decrease the power of linkage dramatically. Large case-control association studies are the method of choice to identify these loci. However, those studies require a lot of prior knowledge about human genome and gene structures and also require systematic screening for polymorphisms in the genes of interest and functional studies of genes and the whole signaling pathway before genetic studies can be targeted and meaningful.

Role of population selection when complex disorders are mapped

In the oligogenic model of inheritance, the major difficulty in gene-mapping studies using linkage is how to avoid locus heterogeneity between the families. In other words, how do we identify the families in which the molecular-genetic background of asthma is similar? Therefore, one way to approach this issue is a careful selection of the study population. If asthma is assumed to be an oligogenic disease at patient level (Figs. 2A and 3), selecting patients who belong to the same large pedigree and share their ancestry is the most efficient way to achieve genetic homogeneity among the patients. This approach is possible in young founder populations in which a small number of unrelated founders has expanded in isolation to a size from which an adequate sample size can be collected. The present-day patients can be considered offspring of only few pedigrees, even if precise genealogical ties between the patients are not known (Fig. 5). In these populations, the gene-mapping strategy can be optimized and the impact of uncertainties in the disease model minimized.

While the benefits of genetic homogeneity (a major mutation among the patients and wider intervals of linkage disequilibrium) in founder populations have been clearly established in rare, monogenetic disorders, their role in common, multifactorial diseases is not clear [28, 29]. Based on simulated data, it has been argued that the populations, which have been useful for identifying rare Mendelian disorders, might not be homogeneous enough for gene-mapping studies in common diseases [30]. The more frequent the susceptibility alleles are in the host population, the fewer the number of settlers (a narrow genetic bottleneck) must be in order to allow expansion of only one (or few) susceptibility-allele-carrying chromosome after separation (Fig. 6). Therefore, the number of unrelated founding chromosomes has to be significantly smaller in common diseases than in rare diseases in order to benefit

11

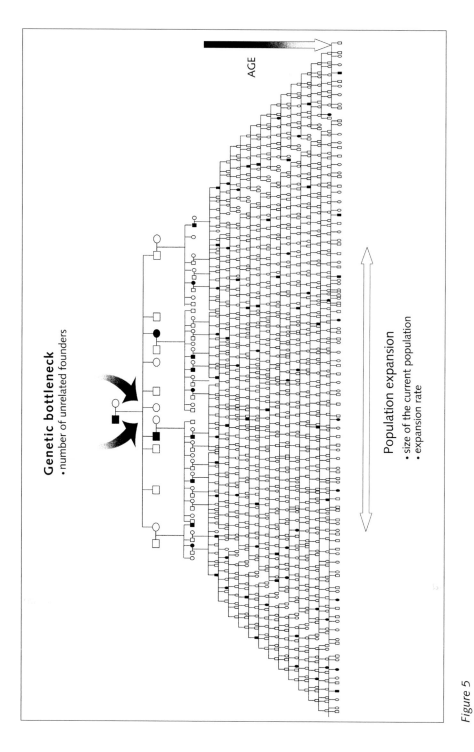

Figure 5
Characteristics of the population history significant for genetic homogeneity and linkage disequilibrium.

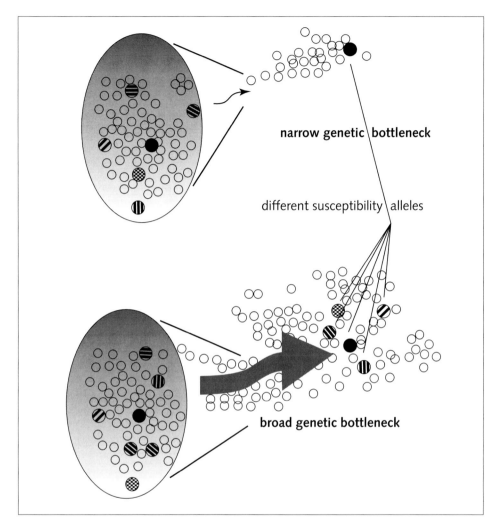

Figure 6
When common disorders such as asthma are studied, the genetic bottleneck has to be narrower than in rare diseases to benefit the genetic homogeneity of the population.

from genetic homogeneity among patients. It has been hypothesized that the number of founders has be as low as a couple of hundred in common disorders such as asthma [17].

Asthma has been studied in several founder populations, including the Finns [31]. Based on the above-mentioned hypothesis, the Finns as a whole are genetically too heterogeneous to be beneficial in genetic studies of such a common disease as asthma. However, regional sub-isolates found in the so-called late-settlement region of Finland are known to fulfill the criteria of a small breeding unit and can offer unique circumstances for gene-mapping studies. After Finland was permanently inhabited about 2000 years ago, the population remained for centuries small and isolated in the coastal regions, which still today are the most densely populated areas in Finland (early settlement). During the 16th century, the rest of the country was slowly settled by internal migration (late settlement). For political and economical reasons, this internal migration was initiated almost exclusively by settlers from one province. Once the settlements of 40 to 60 founding families were established, they again grew in isolation. Rapid expansion of the population did not start until in the beginning of the 18th century, which led to enrichments of several disease genes into these regional isolates. In many recessive diseases, the molecule-genetic studies have found a major mutation among the patients, and in some cases, using the parish records, the common ancestor have been identified [32]. Some multifactorial disorders, such as schizophrenia, multiple sclerosis, and diabetes type II, have found to cluster into the late-settlement regions of Finland [29]. In asthma, a genome-wide scan showed significant evidence for one major susceptibility locus among the patients who originated in one of these late-settlement sub-isolates [33]. However, until the individual susceptibility genes and their disease-associated polymorphims have been described in asthma or other multifactorial diseases, it is difficult say which benefits these populations can offer in the identification of disease genes.

If we assume that asthma is multigenetic disorder at the family and patient level (Figs. 2B and 3), the traditional linkage studies in mixed or founder populations are most likely not going to be more helpful than mixed populations. Identification of minor loci that become of importance by being frequent in the population demand large patient case-control association studies. The founder populations described above are usually rather small in size, which restricts the possibility of collecting the large sample sizes needed, especially if certain allele combinations, e.g., the polymorphisms in gene of a particular signaling pathway, are studied simultaneously. However, these kinds of studies will become possible and more reasonable in the near future together with our increasing knowledge of human genome, gene structures and coding polymorphisms, and more cost-efficient genotyping methods. Since both modes of inheritance are possible in asthma, different study approaches and study populations are also needed in the future studies.

Acknowledgements
I would like to thank professor Juha Kere for his valuable comments on the manuscript.

References

1   Jenkins MA, Hopper JL, Giles GG (1997) Regressive logistic modeling of familial aggregation for asthma in 7,394 population-based nuclear families. *Genet Epidemiol* 14: 317–332

2   Laitinen T, Räsänen M, Kaprio J, Koskenvuo M, Laitinen LA (1998) Importance of genetic factors in adolescent asthma – A population based twin-family study. *Am J Respir Crit Care Med* 157: 1–6

3   Vyse TJ, Todd JA (1996) Genetic analysis of autoimmune disease. *Cell* 85: 311–318

4   Lichtenstein P, Svartengren M. (1997) Genes, environments, and sex: factors of importance in atopic diseases in 7–9-year-old Swedish twins. *Allergy* 52: 1079–1086

5   Harris JR, Magnus P, Samuelsen SO, Tambs K (1997) No evidence for effects of family environment on asthma. A retrospective study of Norwegian twins. *Am J Resp Crit Care Med* 156: 43–49

6   Skadhauge LR, Christiansen K, Kyvik KO, Sigsgaard T (1999) Genetic and environmental influence on asthma: a population-based study of 11,688 Danish twin pairs. *Eur Resp J* 13: 8–14

7   Nieminen MM, Kaprio J, Koskenvuo M (1991) A population-based study of bronchial asthma in adult twin pairs. *Chest* 100: 70–75

8   Edfors-Lubs ML (1971) Allergy in 7000 twin pairs. *Acta Allergologica* 26: 249–285

9   Larsen FS, Holm NV, Henningsen K (1986) Atopic dermatitis. A genetic-epidemiologic study in a population-based twin sample. *J Am Acad Dermat* 15: 487–494

10 Räsänen M, Laitinen T, Kaprio J, Koskenvuo M, Laitinen LA (1998) Hay fever – A nationwide study of adolescent twins and their parents. *Allergy* 53: 885–890

11 Los H, Koppelman GH, Postma DS (1999) The importance of genetic influences in asthma. *Eur Resp J* 14: 1210–1227

12 Palmer LJ, Cookson WO (2000) Genomic approaches to understanding asthma. *Genome Res* 10: 1280–1287

13 Palmer LJ, Burton PR, James AL, Musk AW, Cookson WO (2000) Familial aggregation and heritability of asthma-associated quantitative traits in a population-based sample of nuclear families. *Eur J Hum Genet* 11: 853–860

14 Becker KG, Simon RM, Bailey-Wilson JE, Freidlin B, Biddison WE, McFarland HF, Trent JM (1998) Clustering of non-major histocompatibility complex susceptibility candidate loci in human autoimmune diseases. *Proc Natl Acad Sci USA* 95: 9979–9984

15 Huopio H, Reimann F, Ashfield R, Komulainen J, Lenko HL, Rahier J, Vauhkonen I, Kere J, Laakso M, Ashcroft F et al. (2000) Dominantly inherited hyperinsulinism caused by a mutation in the sulfonylurea receptor type 1. *J Clin Invest* 106: 897–906

16 Thomson JR, Machado RD, Pauciulo MW, Morgan NV, Humbert M, Elliott GC, Ward K, Yacoub M, Mikhail G, Rogers P et al. (2000) Sporadic primary pulmonary hypertension is associated with germline mutations of the gene encoding BMPR-II, a receptor member of the TGF-beta family. *J Med Genet* 37: 741–745

17 Kruglyak L (1999) Prospects for whole-genome linkage disequilibrium mapping of common disease genes. *Nature Genet* 22: 139–144

18   Collins FS, Guyer MS, Charkravarti A (1997) Variation on a theme: cataloguing human DNA sequence variation. *Science* 278: 1580–1581

19   Daniels SE, Bhattacharrya S, James A, Leaves NI, Young A, Hill MR, Faux JA, Ryan GF, le Souef PN, Lathrop GM et al (1996) A genome-wide search for quantitative trait loci underlying asthma. *Nature* 383: 247–250

20   The Collaborative Study on the Genetics of Asthma (1997) A genome-wide search for asthma susceptibility loci in ethnically diverse populations. *Nature Genet* 15: 389–392

21   Ober C, Cox NJ, Abney M, Di Rienzo A, Lander ES, Changyaleket B, Gidley H, Kurtz B, Lee J, Nance M et al (1998) Genome-wide search for asthma susceptibility loci in a founder population. *Hum Mol Genet* 7: 1393–1398

22   Wjst M, Fischer G, Immervoll T, Jung M, Saar K, Rueschendorf F, Reis A, Ulbrecht M, Gomolka M, Weiss EH et al (1999) A genome-wide search for linkage to asthma. *Genomics* 58: 1–8

23   Ober C, Tsalenko A, Parry R, Cox NJ (2000) A second-generation genomewide screen for asthma-susceptibility alleles in a founder population. *Am J Hum Genet* 67: 1154–1162

24   Xu J, Postma DS, Howard TD, Koppelman GH, Zheng SL, Stine OC, Bleecker ER, Meyers DA (2000) Major genes regulating total serum immunoglobulin E levels in families with asthma. *Am J Hum Genet* 67: 1163–1173

25   De Breakeleer M, Ferec C (1996) Mutations in the cystic fibrosis gene in men with congenital bilateral absence of the vas deferens. *Hum Mol Reprod* 2: 669–677

26   Richard G, Smith LE, Bailey RA, Itin P, Hohl D, Epstein EH Jr, DiGiovanna JJ, Compton JG, Bale SJ (1998) Mutations in the human connexin gene GJB3 cause erythrokeratodermia variabilis. Nature Genet 20: 366–369

27   Xia JH, Liu CY, Tang BS, Pan Q, Huang L, Dai HP, Zhang BR, Xie W, Hu DX, Zheng D et al (1998) Mutations in the gene encoding gap junction protein beta-3 associated with autosomal dominant hearing impairment. *Nature Genet* 20: 370–373

28   Peltonen L, Palotie A, Lange K (2000) Use of population isolates for mapping complex traits. *Nature Rev Genet* 1: 182–190

29   Kere J (2001) Human population genetics: lessons from Finland. *Annual Rev Genomics Hum Genet* 2: 103–128

30   Wright AF, Carothers AD, Pirastu M (1999) Population choice in mapping genes for complex diseases. *Nature Genet* 23: 397–404

31   Kauppi P, Laitinen LA, Laitinen H, Kere J, Laitinen T (1998) Verification of self-reported asthma and allergy in subjects and in their family members volunteering for gene mapping studies. *Resp Med* 92: 1281–1288

32   Vuorio AF, Turtola H, Piilahti KM, Repo P, Kanninen T, Kontula K (1997) Familial hypercholesterolemia in the Finnish north Karelia. A molecular, clinical, and genealogical study. *Arterioscler Thromb Vasc Biol* 17: 3127–2138

33   Laitinen T, Daly MJ, Rioux JD, Kauppi P, Laprise C, Petäys T, Green T, Cargill M, Haantela T, Lander ES et al (2001) A susceptibility locus for asthma-related traits on chromosome 7 revealed by genome-wide scan in a founder population. *Nature Genet* 28: 87–91

Genome scans for asthma

Matthias Wjst

Gruppe Molekulare Epidemiologie, Institut für Epidemiologie, GSF – Forschungszentrum für Umwelt und Gesundheit, Ingolstädter Landstrasse 1, D-85758 Neuherberg/Munich, Germany

Introduction

In 1989 highly variable DNA repeats were described as short tandem repeats of a few base pairs (bps) [1]. The repeated elements are usually di-, tri-, or tetranucleotide sequences ($[CA]_n$, $[CAG]_n$, or $[AGAT]_n$). The number of elements in these blocks is variable and ranges between 10 and 100. The evolutionary reasons for these microsatellites, as they have been immediately termed, are not fully understood. They are probably a side-effect of DNA replication, wherein a gap by polymerase slippage is filled by additional bases. The term "microsatellite DNA" derives from the initial observation of these repeats as side or satellite bands by ultracentrifugation over a CsCl density gradient. Even though there are no known biological functions, two distinct features make the microsatellites interesting. First, they are more or less evenly distributed over the whole human genome. The most common microsatellite is the dinucleotide $[CA]_n$ repeat, which comprises around 0.5% of the human genome, making up to 50,000 microsatellites likely. The 1996 Généthon map gives the location of more than 5000 dinucleotide repeats with an average heterozygosity of 70%. The second interesting characteristic of the microsatellites is their variable repeat length between individuals that can be easily measured as length of the sequence amplified by polymerase chain reaction (PCR) between primers flanking the repeat region. Tri- and tetranucleotide repeats are around 10% less common than dinucleotide repeats but have the advantage of being more stable during PCR and easier to score on systems using fluorescent primers and automated detectors.

Linkage analysis

The repeat length ("allele") is inherited in a codominant manner, making it possible to use microsatellites as markers of chromatide segments that were recombined during meiosis. If two children are affected by the same disease and also share the same microsatellite marker allele, it is likely that they have inherited the gene in the proximity of this microsatellite marker ("linkage"). In the next step, it must be determined in a larger number of families whether the sharing of a common segment occurs more often than expected by chance. This approach to localize genes in the genome without any prior knowledge has been called positional cloning [2]. Although suggested in a seminal paper by Botstein as early as 1974 [3], this strategy became feasible only a few years ago.

This approach has been applied successfully to a large number of monogenic diseases, such as Duchenne muscular dystrophy, retinoblastoma, and cystic fibrosis. It seems therefore promising that genes for a complex disease like asthma can be mapped in a similar way. There are, however, some caveats: because the expression of genes in complex diseases is highly influenced by enviromental conditions, a sufficiently high environmental exposure will be necessary. Furthermore, since the number of genes and their relative effects are unknown, the number of families will probably be much higher than for the analysis of a strong, single-gene effect. Finally, because complex diseases are difficult to define, all attempts will have to be made to exclude phenocopies from the same study.

Recombination takes place during meiosis, wherein different grandparents contribute different chromosomal fragments that may be either recombinant or nonrecombinant [4]. The extent of genetic linkage is measured by the recombination fraction. A frequency, for example, of 10 recombinations during 100 meiosis is said to be 10 centiMorgan (cM) apart. The typing of several markers gives the opportunity to construct an ordered genetic map from the recombination frequency between two given markers. These maps do not translate directly into physical maps, as the frequency of recombination events is not distributed evenly over the genome. However, as a rule of thumb, 1 cM is equivalent to 1 million bps, which will harbor an average of 50 genes.

Linkage of two marker is usually assumed when the probability for linkage as opposed to the probability against linkage is greater than the ratio $10^3:1$. The logarithm of this ratio (odds) is called the LOD score, where a LOD score of 3 corresponds to an odds ratio of 1000:1. As in genome scans, a problem with multiple testing arises, and threshold values have been suggested that define a critical limit for allele sharing methods in humans. $p < 7.4 \times 10^{-4}$ (LOD 2.2) is thought to be suggestive for linkage and $p < 2.2 \times 10^{-5}$ (LOD 3.6) as being linked [5]. These theoretical considerations will have to be balanced with practical study limitations like a finite number of families or laboratory resources. It is therefore still an unsolved question how to avoid false-positive linkage claims while at the same time taking into consideration that an overly cautious approach runs the risk of missing true linkages [6]. In contrast, the demand for replication and extension of linkage studies is generally accepted.

Genome scans in humans

Starting with linkage studies in selected candidate regions [7, 8] it soon became obvious that only a more systematic approach would be succesful to find all chromosomal regions associated with asthma [9, 10]. Since 1992 more or less complete marker maps are available for the human genome [11], which has led several groups to start with plans for asthma genome scans.

One of the first asthma studies was perfomed by the Canadian group of Slutsky and Zamel, who examined the whole population of the small island Tristan da Cunha. This population derived from a small number of multi-ethnic founding fathers in 1810. It is a small island of 98 km² with a 2060 m peak where islanders live in a small settlement. Clinical data could be obtained from 282 subjects in October 1993 [12]. Using 270 markers, two distinct loci, "*wheez1*" and "*wheez2*", with strong linkage ($p < 0.00001$) could be identified [13]. The exact position of the linkages, however, has not been released [14].

The first study was published in 1996 by Daniels et al. [15] and examined one qualitative (atopy) and four quantititative traits (IgE, skin prick test index, eosinophil count, dose-response slope of the methacholine provocation). The first group of 80 Australian families included 172 sib pairs with a mean age of the children of 12 years. A second sample of 77 nuclear and extended families including 268 sib pairs was recruited from clinics in Great Britain. All were screened with 269 markers (16 of these on the X chromosome), giving evidence of 6 potential linkages at a $p < 0.001$ level on chromosome 4, 6, 7, 11, 13, and 16. Because only 12% of the study participants had asthma [16], Table 1 gives the results only for atopy or asthma.

The second study was published one year later by examining the phenotype asthma in 43 African American, 79 Caucasian, and 18 Hispanic families with 380 affected individuals that were tested by 360 tetranucleotide markers [16]. Children were of approximately the same age as in the British study. In 70–87% of the study participants, at least one skin test was positive. The lowest p-value for linkage was 0.0005 on 2q33 in Hispanics with different results in the different ethnic groups: 5p15 and 17p11 in African Americans, 11p15 and 19q13 in white Americans, and 2q33 and 21q21 in Americans of Hispanic origin. Furthermore the regions 5q23, 6p21, 12q14, 13q21, and 14q11 have all been described as linked to asthma. A later analysis of the sensitivity to the allergen *D. pteronyssinus* showed two more regions on 2q21 and 8p23 [17] in addition to 6p21 [18].

These results correspond only partially with the results of an inbred population of Hutterites [19]. The Hutterites originated from less than 90 ancestors in Austria and migrated to South Dakota in the U.S. in the 1870s. With a population of approx 35,000, they now live on communal farms. A genome-wide scan was performed in 653 subjects with a mean age between 25 and 30. They were divided into a primary and replication sample, with 292 autosmal and 3 XY pseudoautosomal markers

Table 1 - Probability (p-value) for linkage in genome-wide scans

Chromo-some	Marker	Distance (cM)	Daniels & Bhattacharrya Allergy or asthma	CSGA Asthma	Wjst Asthma	Ober Asthma (loose or strict)
1	D1S228	33.2			0.0406	
	D1S2134	71.9				0.0349
	D1S495	143.1				0.0104
	D1S238	208.9	< 0.05			
	D1S549	244.1				0.0234
	D1S235	260.3	< 0.05			
2	interpolated	47.3		0.0234		
	D2S2298	67.8			**0.0073**	
	D2S1334	173.5				0.0116
	interpolated	231.5		**0.0010**		
	D2S125	266.5	< 0.01			0.0191
3	D3S1744	168.6				0.0197
4	D4S405	57.5				0.0291
	D4S398	74.1	< 0.01			
	D4S430	125.1	< 0.05			
	interpolated	162.5		0.0364		
	D4S2368	167.8				0.0143
	D4S1535	199.0			0.0394	
	D4S426	211.1	< 0.05			
5	interpolated	18.2		0.0016		
	D5S426	51.7				0.0184
	D5S418	58.8			0.0300	
	interpolated	125.7		**0.0375**		
	D5S1480	158.7				**0.0126**
6	D6S309	12.8			0.0134	
	D6S1281	38.5				0.0067
	interpolated	44.12		**0.0263**		
	D6S291	49.8	< 0.01		**0.0081**	
	HLA-Dp1	± 50.0				0.0237
	D6S308	144.1	< 0.05			
7	D7S517	6.1			0.0254	
	D7S1802	24.7				0.0184
	D7S528	58.3			0.0255	
	interpolated	108.8		0.0496		
	D7S1804	132.5				0.0186

Table 1 (continued)

Chromo-some	Marker	Distance (cM)	Daniels & Bhattacharrya Allergy or asthma	CSGA Asthma	Wjst Asthma	Ober Asthma (loose or strict)
8	D8S261	37.7			0.0469	
	D8S298	43.4				0.0124
	interpolated	94.0		0.0411		
	interpolated	146.1		0.0318		
9	IFNA	18.0				0.0374
	D9S156	29.4			0.0109	
	D9S15	84.9	< 0.05			
	D9S910	99.0				0.0237
	D9S1784	112.5			**0.0073**	
10	D10SS674	38.7				0.0291
	D10S1223	160.4				0.0339
	D10S212	179.8			0.0401	
11	D11S2362	5.0				0.0349
	interpolated	23.2		**0.0178**		
	FcεR1β	71.2	< 0.00001			
	D11S1369	76.5				0.0197
	interpolated	123.6		0.0344		
	D11S968	149.7			0.0411	
12	D12S391	19.6				0.0390
	interpolated	45.6		0.0323		
	D12S90	72.3				**0.0143**
	interpolated	93.7		**0.0082**		
	D12S351	97.0			**0.0103**	
13	D13D1493	19.0				0.0126
	D13S153	43.4	< 0.001			
	D13S274	87.7	< 0.05			
	D13S285	108.7				0.0197
	interpolated	111.0		**0.0033**		
14	interpolated	15.2		**0.0124**		
15	interpolated	61.3		0.0464		
	D15S205	72.0			0.0423	
	D15S127	79.4	< 0.05			
16	D16S420	39.2	< 0.05			
	D16S289	90.5	< 0.001			

Table 1 (continued)

Chromo-some	Marker	Distance (cM)	Daniels & Bhattacharrya Allergy or asthma	CSGA Asthma	Wjst Asthma	Ober Asthma (loose or strict)
17	interpolated	2.9		0.0165		
	interpolated	70.3		**0.0030**		
	D17S784	117.1				0.0411
18	D18S851	83.2				0.0455
19	interpolated	9.8		0.0038		
	interpolated	60.1		**0.0026**		
	D19S246	60.8				**0.0027**
20	D20S1085	96.7				0.0497
21	D21S1256	8.6			0.0383	
	D21S1440	31.9				**0.0325**
	interpolated	38.2		**0.0079**		
22	D22S683	34.5				0.0143
	PDGFβ	67.0	< 0.05			

Bold: Marked as significant in the primary publication.
Gray background: p < 0.05 in at least 3 of 4 studies within the same linkage region.
The table relies on the directly submitted results. Differences from the results reported in the original papers are explained by
- recalculation of LOD scores as p values and using a uniform significance limit of p < 0.05;
- minor differences of submitted and published values;
- restriction to loci within an approximately 30 cM interval with the strongest effect;
- neglect of results in subgroups, e.g., including only the strongest effect of all examined populations in the CSGA study;
- exclusion of markers that could not be assigned on the Généthon linkage map of 1995 or being supplemented by GDB entries at time of publication;
- restriction to the phenotype asthma.

showing linkage to asthma in 12 regions. Markers on the regions 5q23-31, 12q15-24.1, 19q13, and 21q21 showed possible linkage in both samples, with the lowest p-value being 0.0009 for the "loose" asthma definition.

In our own study of 97 families with 156 asthma sib pairs, we used a panel of 351 markers with 18 markers located on the X chromosome. 86% of the families had German nationality and the median age of the children was 10 years. Of the phenotypes examined initially (asthma, bronchial hyperreactivity, peak flow variation, total IgE, any sepcific IgE and eosinophil count) the traits asthma and total IgE showed identical linkages on chromosomes 2, 6, 9, and 12, with the lowest *p*-value being 0.0073 [20]. Results for specific IgE were scattered across the genome, with a maximum linkage for *D. pteronyssinus* at D1S21, mixed grass at D5S419, birch at D11S902, and cat at D12S85, which makes it likely that these are spurious linkages [21].

Further asthma[1] genome scans are currently being done by groups in France (M.-H. Dizier), Iceland (H. Hakonarson, Decode Genetics), The Netherlands (D. Postma), Italy (P. Pignatti), Denmark (A. Haagerup), Japan (Y. Yokouchi), and China (S. Weiss). The French data have been presented in abstract form with replicated linkages on chromosomes 1p, 12q, and 17q [22], while the Dutch group assigned linkage to chromosomes 1 to 7, 12, 14, 16, and 17 for asthma-associated traits [23]. Results presented here are therefore preliminary. It is expected that these forthcoming studies will contribute evidence for specific linkage positions that could considerably change the current asthma genome map.

Genome scans in the mouse

Many animal models have been developed that carry asthma-like phenotypes [9]. A first genome-wide scan in the mouse measured acetylcholine airway sensitivity in a body plethysmograph [25]. Three loci were found that have their human homologues on chromosomes 20, 21, and 22. A second study examined ovalbumin-induced bronchoconstriction and described five linked loci with corresponding regions in human chromosomes 5q31, 6p21, 11q23, 12q22, and 17q12 [26]. Interestingly, most of these linkages are in accordance with linkages that have been already described in the human studies.

Interpretion issues

Table 1 compares the first four human-genome scans data side by side. Several points, in addition to the technical remarks in the table legend, make this comparison difficult:

- Families have been selected by different diagnostic criteria. This makes it possible that there are different prevailing asthma sub-types between the studies [21].

---

1 Partially associated to asthma could be familial eosinophilia, an autosomal dominant disorder that has been mapped in a large U.S. kindred to 5q31 with a multipoint LOD score of 6.49 [24].

As a consequence, the replication will not always be possible in another study. Because asthma seems to be a complex syndrome from a clinical view, more information is necessary to differentiate clinical sub-types (extrinsic/ intrinisc, early/late onset), primary trigger types, and severity grades to solve the genetic heterogeneity. Phenotypic pleiotropy is also possible but is not expected to be a major problem during the gene-discovery process.

- Marker characteristics (position, polymorphismus information content, genotype numbers) and clinical examination (type of examination, validity, accuracy, reproducibility) are different in these studies. An exact one-to-one comparison is therefore not possible, even for the phenotype asthma that has been defined in a distinguished manner.

- It is not clear how far away a marker can be located in opposition to a gene and still be considered linked. A simulation using the multipoint LOD curve for an entire chromosome showed a standard error of 7.9 cM and a 95% confidence interval for the replication of a linked gene in the same 31.1 cM area. The standard error of 7.9 cM corresponds to the expected LOD score of about 1.0 or $p = 0.0319$ and falls with increasing LOD scores [27]. A denser marker set in the linked regions will at least be necessary in order to define the exact overlap between studies.

- Observed minor effects such as a preferentially maternal inheritance will have to be examined in more detail, as these effects could considerably change the presented LODs.

- Family numbers and significance values required by statistical simulations have not been reached in the present studies. It is therefore necessary to use larger sample sizes [28].

- None of the studies included detailed information on previous environmental exposure to air pollution, allergens, and respiratory infections. This information, however, is critical to the detection of underlying genetic effects.

- Finally, because asthma is associated with many different other traits like bronchial hyperreactivity or high IgE levels, it is not clear whether asthma genes have been mapped in these studies or only genes that are associated with one of the above traits. The analysis of subgroups from large datasets will probably help to separate different gene effects.

Taking these precautions into account, it is still likely that these first four studies have identified regions for asthma genes. Four linkage regions are found by at least three studies: chromosomes 2 proximal to marker D2S125, 6 at D6S291, 12 proximal to D12S351, and 13 at D13S285. However, regions on chromosomes 5 and 11 are also very promising candidate regions at the moment.

Future prospects

The further refining of the linkage map down to 1 or 2 cM is possible by examination of linkage disequilibrium, the non-random association with alleles of neighboring polymorphisms [29]. However, finding all genes is still a difficult enterprise. From research into other complex diseases like diabetes, coronary heart disease, or schizophrenia, it is evident that the current positional cloning strategy still poses a major hurdle between the linkage region and the gene of interest. As can be seen in the other chapters, most groups are focusing on the sequence variation in functional candidate genes of these linked regions. While this strategy may indeed be succesful in one or more instances, the systematic method of positional cloning by genome scans is being abandoned.

To narrow down the search, attempts at chromosome microdissection and cosmid walking have been done in the past, which can be done now much more efficiently by using yeast artificial chromosomes (YACs). If the gene of interest is large enough, the disease allele could be found if it contains a larger insertion, deletion, or translocation that is detectable by pulsed field gel electrophoresis (PFGE) of DNA. Even if the disease allele, as is expected for asthma, consists of more subtle changes like single-base exchanges (single-nucleotide polymorphism (SNP)), the target gene can be found by a modified HPLC.

A possibility is the brute-force sequencing of the whole linkage region in asthma cases and unaffected controls followed by an *in silico* comparison of the sequence variation. Increased conventional sequencing capacities or new methods like hybridization to sample chips could be a way to accomplish this goal. Also promising are alternative methods for finding altered DNA sequences in pooled samples. Independent of these further strategies, however, there is no doubt that the genome scans are the mainstay of the present asthma gene search.

Acknowledgements
I wish to thank B. Cookson, N. Rich, and C. Ober for making the original linkage data available at the Asthma Gene Database (http://cooke.gsf.de) [30].

References

1   Weber JL, May PE (1989) Abundant class of human DNA polymorphisms which can be typed using the polymerase chain reaction. *Am J Hum Genet* 44: 388–396
2   Collins FS (1992) Positional cloning: let's not call it reverse anymore. *Nature Genetics* 1: 3–6
3   Botstein D, White RL, Skolnick M, Davis RW (1980) Construction of a genetic linkage map in man using restriction fragment length polymorphisms. *Am J Hum Genet* 32: 314–331

4   Ott J (1991) *Analysis of human genetic linkage.* Johns Hopkins University Press, Baltimore, MD

5   Lander E, Kruglyak L (1995) Genetic dissection of complex traits: guidelines for interpreting and reporting linkage results. *Nature Genetics* 11: 241–247

6   Morton NE (1998) Significance levels in complex inheritance. *Am J Hum Genet* 62: 690–697 (Published erratum in *Am J Hum Genet* (1998) 63: 1252)

7   Eiberg H, Lind P, Mohr J, Nielsen LS (1985) Linkage relationship between the human immunoglobulin-E polymorphism and marker. *Cytogen Cell Genet* 40: 622

8   Cookson WOCM, Sharp PA, Faux JA, Hopkin JM (1989) Linkage between immunoglobulin E responses underlying asthma and rhinitis and chromosome 11q. *Lancet* 1: 1292–1295

9   Sandford A, Weir T, Pare P (1996) The genetics of asthma. *Am J Respir Crit Care Med* 153: 1749–1765

10   Holloway JW, Beghé B, Holgate ST (1999) The genetic basis of atopic asthma. *Clin Exp Allergy* 29: 1023–1032

11   Weissenbach J, Gyapay G, Dib C, Vignal A, Morissette J, Millasseau P, Vaysseix G, Lathrop M (1992) A second-generation linkage map of the human genome. *Nature* 359: 794–801

12   Zamel N (1995) In search of the genes of asthma on the island of Tristan da Cunha. *Can Respir J* 2: 18–22

13   Holgate ST (1997) Asthma genetics: waiting to exhale. *Nature Genetics* 15: 227–229

14   Vogel G (1997) A scientific result without the science. *Science* 276: 1327

15   Daniels SE, Bhattacharrya S, James A, Leaves NI, Young A, Hill MR, Faux JA, Ryan GF, de LeSoeuf PN, Lathrop GM et al. (1996) A genome-wide search for quantitative trait loci underlying asthma. *Nature* 383: 247–250

16   CSGA. The Collaborative Study on the Genetics of Asthma (1997) A genome-wide search for asthma susceptibility loci in ethnically diverse populations. *Nature Genetics* 15: 389–392

17   Hizawa N, Freidhoff LR, Chiu YF, Ehrlich E, Luehr CA, Anderson JL, Duffy DL, Dunston GM, Weber JL, Huang SK et al (1998) Genetic regulation of *Dermatophagoides pteronyssinus*-specific IgE responsiveness: a genome-wide multipoint linkage analysis in families recruited through 2 asthmatic sibs. Collaborative Study on the Genetics of Asthma (CSGA). *J Allergy Clin Immunol* 102: 436–442

18   Hizawa N, Freidhoff LR, Ehrlich E, Chiu YF, Duffy DL, Schou C, Dunston GM, Beaty TH, Marsh DG, Barnes KC et al (1998) Genetic influences of chromosomes 5q31–q33 and 11q13 on specific IgE responsiveness to common inhaled allergens among African American families. Collaborative Study on the Genetics of Asthma (CSGA). *J Allergy Clin Immunol* 102: 436–442

19   Ober C, Cox NJ, Abney M, di Rienzo A, Lander AS, Changyaleket B, Gidley H, Kurtz B, Lee J, Nance M et al (1998) Genome-wide search for asthma susceptibility loci in a founder population. *Hum Mol Gen* 7: 1393–1398

20   Wjst M, Fischer G, Immervoll T, Jung M, Saar K, Rueschendorf F, Reis A, Ulbrecht M,

Gomolka M, Weiss EH et al (1999) A genome-wide search for linkage to asthma. *Genomics* 58: 1–8

21 Wjst M for the German Asthma Genetics Group (1999) Specific IgE – One gene fits all? *Clin Exp Allergy* 29 (Suppl 4): 5–10

22 Dizier MH, Matran R, Meunier F, Neukirch F, Pacheco Y, Parent V, Paty E, Pin I, Pison C, Scheinmann P et al (1999) Genome screen for asthma and related phenotypes in the French EGEA study. *Am Rev Respir Crit Care Med* 159 (Suppl): A649

23 Koppleman GH, Stine OC, Howard TD et al (1998). Genome screen for asthma susceptibility loci in a restricted Dutch population (abstract). *Am J Hum Gen* 63 (Suppl): 1705

24 Rioux JD, Stone VA, Daly MJ, Cargill M, Green T, Nguyen H, Nutman T, Zimmerman PA, Tucker MA, Hudson T et al (1998) Familial eosinophilia maps to the cytokine gene cluster on human chromosomal region 5q31–q33. *Am J Hum Genet* 63: 1086–1094

25 de Sanctis G, Merchant M, Beier DR, Dredge RD, Grobholz JK, Martin TR, Lander Es, Drazen JM (1995) Quantitative locus analysis of airway hyperresponsivenes in A/J and C57BL/6J mice. *Nature Genetics* 11: 150–154

26 Zhang Y, Lefort J, Kearsley V, Lapa e Silva JR, Cookson WOCM, Vargafting BB (1999) A genome wide search for asthma associated quantitative trait loci in a mouse model of allergic asthma. *Hum Mol Genet* 8: 601–605

27 Roberts SB, MacLean CJ, Neale MC, Eaves LJ, Kendler KS (1999) Replication of linkage studies of complex traits: An examination of variation in location estimates. *Am J Hum Gen* 65: 876–884

28 Todd JA (1999) Interpretation of results from genetic studies of multifactorial diseases. *Lancet* 354 (Suppl 1): 15–16

29 Cookson WOCM (1999). The alliance of genes and environment in asthma and allergy. *Nature* 402 (Suppl): B5–B11

30 Wjst M, Immervoll T (1998) An internet linkage and mutation database for the complex phenotype asthma. *Bioinformatics* 14: 827–828

The role of founder populations in mapping complex disease genes: Studies in the South Dakota Hutterites

Carole Ober

Department of Human Genetics, The University of Chicago, 920 East 58th Street, Room 507C, Chicago, IL 60627, USA

Introduction

Founder populations are populations that are derived from a well-defined ancestral population with little admixture since their founding. Founder populations can be old and derived from a larger number of ancestors, such as the Finnish, Icelandic, Ashkenazi, and Sardinian populations, or young and derived from a much smaller number of founders, such as the Amish, Hutterites, and Tristan de Cunhans [1]. The latter group of founder populations is also inbred, i.e., the inbreeding coefficient is > 0 for nearly everyone in the population because all matings are consanguineous.

There are two recognized advantages of using founder populations for complex trait mapping. First, the finite founder gene pool increases the likelihood that fewer susceptibility alleles (and perhaps fewer loci) will be segregating in the population. As a result, there is presumed to be less genetic heterogeneity associated with any particular phenotype in such populations, making it easier to detect both linkage and association. Second, the younger age of these populations (as compared with non-founder populations) results in fewer meioses since the founding and therefore greater linkage disequilibrium will exist between alleles at linked loci in founder populations than in non-founder populations [2, 3]. This allows for novel strategies that can facilitate gene mapping. Recently, however, it has been suggested by both theoretical and empirical studies that linkage disequilibrium may not extend far enough in older founder populations to be useful for linkage disequilibrium mapping of complex traits [4–6]. On the other hand, the extensive linkage disequilibrium expected to be present in recent founder populations may preclude the fine localization of a disease gene. Therefore, both older and younger founder populations, as well as non-founder populations, will be useful for mapping and positional cloning studies and will provide complementary information regarding the initial localization and eventual identification of asthma genes.

The Hereditary Basis of Allergic Diseases, edited by Stephen T. Holgate and John W. Holloway
© 2002 Birkhäuser Verlag Basel/Switzerland

A potential disadvantage of studies in founder populations is that these populations may harbor "private" mutations that are present only in that particular population. While this is certainly true for single-gene, Mendelian disorders (for examples, see [7–9]), it is much less likely for common diseases with complex patterns of transmission. This is because genetic polymorphisms that influence susceptibility to complex diseases appear to be common variants, such as the Apoε4 allele and coronary heart disease [10], human leukocyte antigens (HLA) alleles and autoimmune diseases [11], variants at the methylene tetrahydrofolate reductase (*MTHFR*) locus and arterial disease [12], and calpain 10 (*CPN10*) variants and type 2 diabetes mellitus [13]. Because common polymorphisms usually are represented in most human populations [14], including founder populations [15], it is likely that common alleles that are associated with common diseases in founder populations would also be present in outbred populations. Thus, while a small founding gene pool may result in reduced heterogeneity in the population (i.e., fewer susceptibility alleles and loci segregating in the population), the susceptibility loci that are present in founder populations will likely be present in larger outbred populations, as we have found in our genetic studies of asthma in the Hutterites [16–19].

The Hutterites of South Dakota

The Hutterites are among the best-characterized young founder populations. The more than 35,000 Hutterites that live in the northern United States and western Canada are derived from fewer than 90 ancestors that lived in Europe from the early 1700s to the early 1800s [20]. The genealogical relationships between all living Hutterites and their relationships to each of the founders are known and documented, as a result of the pioneering genetic-epidemiologic studies of the Hutterites initiated by Dr. Arthur Steinberg and his students in the 1950s and 1960s [21].

The Hutterites of South Dakota, the subjects of our studies, are descendents of only 64 of the original founders. No one has joined the community since they migrated to the United States in the 1870s. Today, the average coefficient of kinship in the population is 0.034 (± 0.015) [22], approximately equivalent to that of first cousins once removed. However, because we do not know the relationship among all 64 founders, and because some may have been related to each other, this may be an underestimate of the true relatedness in the population, as previously discussed [23]. The relative genetic homogeneity of the Hutterites is further reflected in the fact that there are only 15 surnames and that only 12 are represented in the South Dakota Hutterites. In fact, the Hutterites are among the most inbred population of European descent. The restricted gene pool ensures that fewer alleles overall will be segregating in the population and that Hutterites with asthma will be more likely to have asthma because of the same constellation of genes, than are individuals drawn from the general population.

A second feature of the Hutterite population that makes them particularly amenable to genetic studies of complex diseases is that they practice a communal lifestyle. Approximately 10 to15 families live on large communal farms, which are called colonies. Although families have their own houses on the colony, all meals are prepared in a common kitchen and eaten in a communal dining room. The diets are not only uniform from colony to colony but have also changed little over time. Overall, lifestyle factors and environmental exposures are very similar within and between Hutterite colonies (for more details regarding Hutterite lifestyle, see [24]). The relative homogeneity of the Hutterite environment minimizes the effects of non-genetic factors on the differences between individuals with respect to disease, and perhaps even enhances the effects of genes on disease expression.

Genetic studies of asthma and atopy in the Hutterites

Between 1994 and 1997 we studied Hutterites living in nine colonies in South Dakota. All individuals over the age of 5 years and who were home on the days of our visit participated in these investigations. We evaluated all subjects, following the protocol of the Collaborative Study on the Genetics of Asthma (CSGA) [25, 26], with slight modifications. These protocols have been described in detail previously [15, 16, 27]. Our final sample included 693 individuals. The mean age of the participants is 28.7 years (s.d. 17.0 years; range 6 to 89 years) and the male:female sex ratio is 321:372. The clinical characteristics of our study sample are shown in Table 1. The prevalence of strict asthma (symptoms + bronchial hyperresponsiveness (BHR)) in the Hutterites is 11.6%; an additional 12.2% of individuals had asymptomatic BHR, and 11.1% reported asthma symptoms in the absence of BHR. The prevalence of atopy (assessed by ≥ 1 +SPT) ranges from 41.8% in unaffected individuals to 52.1% in asthmatics.

A genome screen using 386 microsatellite markers was completed, yielding a 9.1 cM map. Subjects were genotyped for 177 additional markers in selected regions of the genome, including polymorphisms in 17 candidate genes [16]. Because of the extensive linkage disequilibrium present in this young founder population [28], we use tests of both linkage [29] and linkage disequilibrium [30] with genome-wide markers. Markers in six chromosomal regions showed evidence of linkage by both tests, with at least one p-value ≤ 0.001: 5p with BHR, 5q with asthma, 8p with asthma, 14q with asthma, 16q with +SPT with mold, and 19q with BHR. Other regions that showed evidence of linkage by one test with p-value ≤ 0.001 were 1p with asthma, 1q with +SPT to cockroach, 2q to +SPT to cockroach and mold, 3p with asthma, 3q with +SPT to mold, 9q with asthma symptoms, 11p with +SPT to molds, 13q with symptoms, 18p with asthma symptoms, and 20q with +SPT to HDM.

Despite the fact that the Hutterites have been reproductively isolated for over 200 years and that they are descendents of only 64 individuals, many of the regions

31

Table 1 - Clinical characteristics of the Hutterite sample by asthma affection status (modified from [16]).

	Unaffected	Symptoms only	BHR[a] only	Symptoms + BHR (strict asthma)
Sample size	414	73	80	71
Mean age (years) (sd)	28.8 (15.5)	31.2 (15.5)	24.7 (19.3)	22.51 (15.9)
Sex ratio (M/F)	0.78	0.92	0.90	1.63
Mean log IgE (IU) (sd)	1.3 (0.7)	1.5 (0.8)	1.5 (0.8)	1.8 (0.8)
% +SPT ≥ 1 allergen	41.8	52.0	50.0	52.1
% +SPT ≥ 2 allergens	22.5	26.0	27.5	32.4
% +SPT HDM[b]	21.3	21.9	32.5	29.6
% +SPT cockroach[c]	19.8	23.3	28.8	19.7
% +SPT molds[d]	9.9	11.0	11.3	16.9
% +SPT pollens/trees[e]	20.0	28.8	18.8	36.6
% +SPT animal danders[f]	6.5	8.2	11.3	12.7

[a]*BHR, bronchial hyperresponsiveness to methacholine;* [b]*house dust mite,* D. pteronyssinus *and* D. farinae; [c]*B. germanica and* P. americana; [d]*A. alternata,* C. herbarum, *and* A. fumigatus; [e]*L. perenne,* A. artemisifolia, A. vulgaris, Q. alba, B. verrucosa; [f]*F. domesticus,* C. familiaris

showing evidence of linkage in the Hutterites have also shown evidence of linkage in genome-wide screens in other samples (Tab. 2). This likely reflects the fact that asthma-susceptibility alleles are common variants in the population, as discussed above.

Genome-wide screens for asthma and atopy-susceptibility alleles have been reported for four population samples in addition to the Hutterites: the Busselton (Australian) population [31], the U.S. CSGA families [25, 32], a German population [33, 34], and a French population [35]. Ten of the regions showing evidence of linkage in the Hutterites also show some evidence of linkage (at $p < 0.01$) to a related phenotype in at least one of these outbred samples (Tab. 2). Remarkably, a 20 cM region on 11p has been linked to asthma or atopy in four of the five samples, and a region on 19q has been linked in three of five population samples. It is not surprising that the Hutterites and another sample from Germany share the most linked regions because the Hutterite population is largely of German ancestry. Taken together, these data implicate loci in 10 genomic regions as having susceptibility alleles that are present in diverse population samples and, perhaps, relatively large effects on asthma or atopic phenotypes. Because linkage disequilibrium is greater in

Table 2 - Regions showing evidence for linkage to asthma, atopy, or related phenotypes in the Hutterites and in one or more other genome screens at p < 0.01 (modified from [16]). A review of all of the regions of overlap between the five genome-wide screens is presented elsewhere [36].

Chrom.	cM from p-ter[a]	Hutterites [16]	Busselton [31]	U.S. CSGA [25, 32]	German [33, 34]	French [35]
1	4–14	Asthma			Spec. IgE	
	30–37	Asthma			Eosinophils	
	139–150	+SPT			IgE, Spec. IgE	
2	186–215	+SPT			IgE	
5	33–52	BHR			Spec. IgE	
9	95–112	Symptoms			Asthma	
11	21–43	+SPT		Asthma (Ca)	Spec. IgE	IgE
16	105–125	+SPT	IgE			
19	67–70	BHR		Asthma (Ca)		BHR
20	32–39	+SPT	Wheeze			

[a]Based on the Marshfield map (http://research.marshfieldclinic.org/genetics/)

the Hutterites than in the outbred populations, complementary strategies that take into account the shared linkages in the Hutterites and in outbred populations will facilitate the identification of the susceptibility loci in these linked regions. Such positional cloning strategies are currently underway in our laboratory.

Acknowledgments

The author acknowledges the Hutterites for their enthusiastic participation in these studies and Drs. Rodney Parry and Nancy Cox for their immeasurable contributions to this project. This work was supported by NIH grants HL49596 and HL56399 and the NHLBI Mammalian Genotyping Service (Marshfield, WI).

References

1   Wright AF, Carothers AD, Pirastu M (1999) Population choices in mapping for complex diseases. *Nature Genet* 23: 397–404

2   Lander ES, Schork NJ (1994) Genetic dissection of complex traits. *Science* 265: 2037–2048

3   Ober C, Cox NJ (1998) Mapping genes for complex traits in founder populations. *Clin Exp Allergy* (Supp) 28: 101–105

4   Kruglyak L (1999) Prospects for whole-genome linkage disequilibrium mapping of common disease genes. *Nature Genet* 22: 139–144

5   Eaves IA, Merriman TR, Barber RA, Nutland S, Tuomilehto-Wolf E, Tuomilehto J, Cucca F, Todd JA (2000) The genetically isolated populations of Finland and Sardinia may not be a panacea for linkage disequilibrium mapping of common disease genes. *Nature Genet* 25: 320–323

6   Taillon-Miller P, Bauer-Sardiña I, Saccone NL, Putzel J, Laitinen T, Cao A, Kere J, Pilia G, Rice JP, Kwok P-Y (2000) Juxtaposed regions of extensive and minimal linkage disequilibrium in human Xq25 and Xq28. *Nature Genet* 25: 324–328

7   McKusick VA (1978) *Medical genetic studies of the Amish: selected papers.* Johns Hopkins Univ Press, Baltimore, MD

8   Hostetler JA (1985) History and relevance of the Hutterite population for genetic studies. *Am J Med Genet* 22: 453–462

9   Peltonen L, Jalanko A, Varilo T (1999) Molecular genetics of the Finnish disease heritage. *Hum Mol Genet* 8: 1913–1923

10 Jarvik GP (1997) Genetic predictors of common disease: apolipoprotein E genotype as a paradigm. *Ann Epidemiol* 7: 357–362

11 Lechler R (ed) (1994) *HLA and disease.* Academic Press, Inc, San Diego, CA

12 Arruda VR, von Zuben PM, Chiaparini LC, Annichino-Bizzacchi JM, Costa FF (1997) The mutation Ala677—>Val in the methylene tetrahydrofolate reductase gene: a risk factor for arterial disease and venous thrombosis. *Thromb Haemost* 77: 818–821

13 Horikawa Y, Oda N, Cox NJ, Li X, Hara M, Hinokio Y, Lindner TH, Mashima H, Horikawa Y, Oda Y et al (2000) Polymorphism in the calpain 10 gene affects susceptibility to type 2 diabetes in Mexican Americans. *Nature Genet* 26: 163–175

14 Zietkiewicz E, Yotova V, Jarnik M, Korab-Laskowska M, Kidd KK, Modiano D, Scozzari R, Stoneking M, Tishkoff S, Batzer M et al (1998) Genetic structure of the ancestral population of modern humans. *J Mol Evol* 47: 146–155

15 Ober C, Cox N, Parry R, Abney M, DiRienzo A, Changyaleket B, Gidley H, Kurtz B, Lander ES, Lee J et al (1998) Genome-wide search for asthma susceptibility loci in a founder population. *Hum Molec Genet* 7: 1393–1398

16 Ober C, Tsalenko A, Parry R, Cox NJ (2000) A second generation genome-wide screen for asthma susceptibility alleles in a founder population. *Am J Hum Genet* 67: 1154–1162

17 Ober C, Leavitt SA, Tsalenko A, Howard TD, Hoki DM, Daniel R, Newman DL, Wu X, R. P, Lester LA et al (2000) Variation in the interleukin 4 receptor a gene confers susceptibility to asthma and atopy in ethnically diverse populations. *Am J Hum Genet* 66: 517–526

18 Donfack J, Tsalenko A, Hoki DM, Parry R, Solway J, Lester LA, Ober C (2000) HLA-DRB1*01 alleles and sensitization to cockroach allergies. *JACI* 105: 960–966

19 Summerhill E, Leavitt SA, Gidley H, Parry R, Solway J, Ober C (2000) β2-adrenergic receptor arg16-arg16 genotype is associated with reduced lung function, but not asthma, in the Hutterites. *Am J Resp Crit Care Med* 162: 599–602

20 Martin AO (1970) The founder effect in a human isolate: Evolutionary implications. *Am J Phys Anthropology* 32: 351–368

21 Steinberg AG, Bleibtreu HK, Kurczynski TW, Martin AO, Kurczynski EM (1967) Genetic studies in an inbred human isolate In: JF Crow, JV Neel (eds): *Proceedings of the Third International Congress of Human Genetics*. Johns Hopkins University Press, Baltimore, MD, 267–290

22 Abney MA, McPeek MS, Ober C (2000) Estimation of variance components of quantitative traits in inbred populations. *Am J Hum Genet* 66: 629–650

23 Ober C, Weitkamp LR, Cox N, Dytch H, Kostyu D, Elias S (1997) HLA and mate choice in humans. *Amer J Hum Genet* 61: 497–504

24 Hostetler JA (1974) *Hutterite society*. Johns Hopkins University Press, Baltimore

25 CSGA (1997) A genome-wide search for asthma susceptibility loci in ethnically diverse populations. *Nature Genet* 15: 389–392

26 Lester LA, Ober C, Blumenthal M, Marsh DG, Rich SS, Miller ME, Banks-Schlegel S, Togias A, Bleecker ER, CSGA (2000) Ethnic specific differences in asthma and asthma-associated phenotypes in the collaborative study on the genetics of asthma (CSGA). *JACI* 108: 357–362

27 Ober C, Tsalenko A, Willadsen SA, Newman D, Daniel R, Wu X, Andal J, Hoki D, Schneider D, True K et al (1999) Genome-wide screen for atopy susceptibility alleles in the Hutterites. *Clin Exp Allergy* (Suppl) 4: 11–15

28 Hall D, Cho J, Hill A, Spedini G, Ober C, Di Rienzo A (1997) Comparison of linkage disequilibrium within and between ethnic groups. *Amer J Hum Genet* 61: A200

29 Curtis D, Sham PC (1995) Model-free linkage analysis using likelihoods. *Amer J Hum Genet* 57: 703–716

30 Spielman RS, McGinnis RE, Ewens WJ (1993) Transmission test for linkage disequilibrium: the insulin gene region and insulin dependent diabetes mellitus (IDDM). *Amer J Hum Genet* 52: 506–516

31 Daniels SE, Bhattacharrya S, James A, Leaves NI, Young A, Hills M, Faux J, Ryan G, Le Souef P, Lathrop MG et al (1996) A genome-wide search for quantitative trait loci underlying asthma. *Nature* 383: 247–250

32 Mathias RA, Freidhoff LR, Blumenthal MN, Meyers DA, Lester L, King R, Xu JF, Solway J, Barnes KC, Pierce J et al (2000) A genome-wide linkage analysis of total serum IgE using variance components analysis in asthmatic families. *Genet Epidem* 20: 340–355

33 Wjst M, Fischer G, Immervoll T, Jung M, Saar K, Rueschendorf F, Reis A, Ulbrecht M, Gomolka M, Weiss EH et al (1999) A genome-wide search for linkage to asthma. *Genomics* 58: 1–8

34 Wjst M (1999) Specific IgE – One gene fits all? *Clin Exp Allergy* (Suppl) 4: 5–10

35 Dizier MH, Besse-Schmittler C, Guilloid-Bataille M, Annesi-Maesano I, Boussaha M,

Bousquet J, Charpin D, DeGioanni A, Gormand F, Grimfeld A et al (2000) Genome screen for asthma and related phenotypes in the french EGEA study. *Am J Resp Crit Care Med* 62: 1812–1818

36 Ober C, Moffatt M (2000) Contributing factors to the pathobiology: The genetics of asthma. In: S Wenzel (ed): *The pathobiology of asthma*. W.B. Saunders Company, Philadelphia, PA, 245–261

Genetic regulation of specific IgE responsiveness

Nobuyuki Hizawa

First Department of Medicine, School of Medicine, Hokkaido University, Kita-Ku, N-15 W-7, Sapporo 060-8638, Japan

Introduction

Allergic reactions are the result of specific immunoglobulin E (IgE) antibody production in response to common innocuous antigens. Atopic people are intrinsically prone to produce IgE antibodies against many different allergens. IgE antibody production is driven by antigen-specific Th2 cells that secrete a distinct repertoire of cytokines, including IL-4, IL-5, IL-6, IL-9, and IL-13. Specific IgE responsiveness toward house dust mite (HDM) is associated with asthma and bronchial hyperresponsiveness [1–3]. Specific IgE responses toward allergens derived from cats, dogs, cockroaches, and pollens also contribute significantly to the development of allergic diseases. In particular, a clear correlation was recently demonstrated among cockroach allergy, level of exposure to cockroaches, and asthma-related health problems in inner-city children [4]. Because of the impact that allergies have on public health, it is critical to identify susceptibility factors in the development of specific IgE responses toward common environmental allergens.

Allergic reactions are complex and involve several sets of genes and multiple environmental factors [5, 6]. Segregation analysis of the specific response to allergens (SRA) was performed in a sample of 234 randomly selected Australian families using regressive models [7]. Various SRA phenotypes were considered by using broad and narrow definitions of these phenotypes according to the type of test used, namely skin test or RAST test, and the specificity of the response to allergen. Strong evidence for familial dependency among blood relatives has been demonstrated for most SRA phenotypes. However, the study has failed to find evidence of a Mendelian factor accounting for familial transmission, suggesting that several genes interact with environmental factors to influence the development of specific IgE responses toward common allergens.

The Hereditary Basis of Allergic Diseases, edited by Stephen T. Holgate and John W. Holloway
© 2002 Birkhäuser Verlag Basel/Switzerland

Environmental influences

The importance of environmental factors in the expression of allergies is demonstrated by the relatively low concordance for atopic allergy in monozygotic twin pairs [8]. A strong environmental influence interacting with multiple genetic factors was revealed in a well-defined population with characterized exposure to low-molecular-weight chemicals (ammonium hexa-chloroplatinate (ACP)) [9]. An HLA-DR3 phenotype was found to be more common among specific IgE responders toward ACP (odds ratio [OR] 2.3) and more so in those with low (OR infinite) than with high exposure (OR 1.6). Furthermore, HLA-DR6 was less common among the responders (OR 0.4), and the association was stronger in the low-exposure group (OR 0.1 *versus* 0.5). Significance of exposure levels to mites was also shown on mounting HDM-specific IgE responses in a study that compared exposure levels between HDM-sensitive children and their non-HDM-sensitive atopic siblings [10]. The HDM-sensitive children had significantly higher levels of Der p 1 in their mattresses and bedding. These findings raised the possibility that the development of Th2 cells is influenced by the strength of signals received from antigen-presenting cells (APCs). If the signal is either very low or very high, Th2 cells tend to develop, whereas intermediate signals tend to produce Th1 cells [11].

The increase in the level of industrialization and the number of diesel engines producing diesel exhaust particles (DEP) in the air parallel the increase in allergic airway diseases. Specific IgE responses against pollen grains were measured in Brown Norway (BN) rats sensitized with timothy grass pollen with or without DEP [12]. Specific IgE antibody responses were higher in rats immunized with pollen grains and DEP than in rats immunized with pollen only. The adjuvant activity of DEP found in this model is another example of a strong environmental impact on the development of allergen-specific IgE responses.

Genetic influences

Human leukocyte antigen (HLA)

Much of the interest in genetic control of the immune response to specific allergens has focused on *HLA-D* genes [13]. The complex formed by the HLA class II molecule, a peptide antigen and the T-cell antigen-specific receptor, is essential to trigger antigen specific immune responses, and *HLA-D* genes have been implicated in susceptibility to a wide range of diseases with an immunological basis [14]. A number of studies have shown that specific IgE production toward individual allergens is associated with particular HLA class II alleles [15–18] including Amb a 5, Bet v 1, Lol p 1, and Ole e 1. A study that investigated HLA class II DR and DP associations with IgE responses to six major allergens in a large number of nuclear and extended families recruited through allergy and asthma clinics also showed an association between the HLA-DR allele and IgE responses toward both Fel d I (OR = 2, p = 0.002) and Alt a I (OR = 1.9, p = 0.006) [19].

Marsh et al. found that the HLA-D restriction for IgE response to a short ragweed allergen, Amb a 5, was limited to subjects carrying HLA-DR2 and Dw2 in Caucasians [18, 20]. Using a combination of both DNA sequencing of *HLA-D* genes and human Amb a 5-specific T-cell clones, they clearly established that the HLA-D restriction element is the DR molecule, of which expression is associated with the DR2.2 phenotype [21, 22]. HLA-D restriction in Ag-specific T cells has also been demonstrated in responses to complex allergens such as Der p 1 and Der p 2, major antigenic components of *Dermatophagoides pteronyssinus* [23, 24]. It is, however, important to note that the association between a particular HLA allele and IgE responses to allergens is most striking for low-molecular-weight allergens, which have a relatively limited number of immunodeterminants that are potentially detectable by the immune system. For allergens of intermediate complexity (molecular weight = 10,000 to 20,000), immune recognition may be limited essentially to a single immunodeterminant for subjects with a genetically determined low capacity to synthesize IgE. In the case of very complex allergens such as HDM, genetic regulation of the immune response by *HLA-D* genes is known to be quite complex [5, 25] and to involve multiple epitopes (regions of the allergen that bind to T-cell receptors) and agretopes (regions of the allergen that bind to HLA class II molecule). The major epitope is favored in individuals who have low IgE levels, but all epitopes are potentially recognized in individuals who have high IgE levels [26]. Heterogeneity in HLA class II specificity was demonstrated by recognition of Der p 2 by T cells [27]. Analysis of a panel of Der p 2-specific T-cell clones all isolated from the same HDM-allergic individual revealed the presence of T-cell clones that react with the amino-terminal region of Der p 2 residues 16–31 and 22–40. T-cell recognition of peptide 16–31 was restricted by HLA-DQB1*0301, whereas 22–40 could be presented by both DQB1*0301 and DRB1*1101, illustrating that HLA-DQ and –DR class II molecules of different specificity may function in the presentation of HDM peptides.

The genetic control of specific IgE responsiveness has also been extensively studied in animal models. When serum IgE responses were examined in mice of 12 inbred strains sensitized intraperitoneally with ovalbumin (OVA) and repeatedly exposed to aerosolized OVA, OVA-specific IgE concentrations ranged from less than 3 ng/ml to 455 ng/ml among different strains [28]. This wide difference among inbred mouse strains in the susceptibility to develop specific IgE responsiveness to complex antigens demonstrated that elevation of serum antigen-specific IgE levels is genetically determined. Several studies using different strains of high- and low-responder mice to complex antigens identified a genetic contribution of the *MHC* gene [29, 30]. Another study found that the degree of genetic contribution of *MHC* and non-*MHC* genes to specific IgE responsiveness depended on the amount of antigen administered [31]. A genome-wide search in the Biozzi mice to map relevant genes for antibody responsiveness identified at least eight independently segregating loci responsible for high and low antibody titers when examining IgE antibodies to multi-specific antigens, the strongest of which was the MHC complex [32]. Based on these studies, it is reasonable to hypothesize that the HLA is a necessary, but not sufficient, factor in the development of specific IgE responsiveness to complex allergens, and further genetic and environmental factors appear to be required to determine reactivity to specific allergens.

Interaction between overall IgE-regulating genes and HLA-D genes

The presence of an interaction between IgE-regulating genes and *HLA* genes in the control of certain IgE immune responses has been recognized [33]. Individuals possessing lower total serum IgE levels exhibit significantly higher frequencies of the particular HLA phenotype most strongly associated with responsiveness to the respective allergen. People who exhibit IgE Ab responsiveness to a particular allergen, despite their low capacity for overall IgE responsiveness, apparently require the optimal *HLA* gene to permit the IgE response, whereas this requirement is relaxed in persons having a high capacity to synthesize IgE. Such evidence has been obtained especially in the case of IgE responses toward allergens of intermediate complexity, such as Amb a III, Lol p II, and Lol p III (molecular weight = 10,000 to 15,000) [33, 34].

The immunoblot patterns of specific IgE binding of serum from monozygotic and dizygotic members of a large cohort of Australian twins were examined to determine the extent to which genetic factors control the specificity of IgE responses to individual HDM allergens [35]. HDM proteins separated by sodium dodecyl-sulfate-polyacrylamide gel electrophoresis (SDS-PAGE) were immunoblotted with sera from 317 twin pairs in which at least one twin had at least a weak HDM skin test response. Over all 36 blotted bands, the mean case-wise concordance was 41% for monozygotic twins and 17% for dizygotic twins. Of the components detected, only those with molecular weights of 23 kD and 16 kD were significantly different between the groups ($p < 0.01$). Moreover, in the monozygotic twins, concordance never exceeded 67% for any given band, and most monozygotic individuals recognized components their co-twin did not. These findings suggested that genetic control of overall IgE responsiveness in monozygotic twins is far stronger than that controlling specific sensitization to HDM allergens, and differences observed between the monozygotic and dizygotic twins could be partly explained by overall IgE hyper-responsiveness.

Despite substantial evidence indicating that non-*HLA* genes contribute strongly to the control of specific immune responsiveness [5, 36], little information about the location of these genes is currently available. To clarify this issue, a genome-wide search was conducted for genes controlling specific IgE responsiveness to the Der p allergen [37]. Specific IgE antibody levels to the Der p crude allergen and to the purified allergens Der p 1 and Der p 2 were measured. Multipoint, nonparametric linkage analysis of 370 polymorphic markers was performed using the GENEHUNTER program. The most compelling evidence of genes controlling specific IgE response to Der p was obtained in two novel regions: chromosomes 2q21-q23 (NPL = 2.23; P = 0.0033 for Caucasian subjects) and 8p23-p21 (NPL = 2.05; P = 0.0011 for African American subjects). The interleukin-1 (IL-1) gene cluster that contains IL1A, IL1B, IL17, IL1R and IL18R is located on chromosome 2q21-q23. Also, three regions previously proposed to be candidate regions for atopy, total IgE, or asthma showed evidence of linkage to Der p-specific IgE responsiveness: 6p21 (NPL = 1.72; P = 0.0064) and 13q32-q34 (NPL = 1.72; P = 0.0064) in Caucasian subjects and 5q23-q33 (NPL = 1.28; P = 0.0071) in African American subjects. No single locus, however, generated overwhelming evidence of a linkage in terms of established criteria and guidelines for a genome-wide screening, a finding that supports the notion of a complex etiology for Der p-specific IgE responsiveness.

The German Asthma Genetics Group also conducted a genome-wide quantitative linkage analysis of specific IgE levels to birch, mixed grass, *Dermatophagoides pteronyssinus*, and cat, in which each allergen showed one or two linked regions at different loci [38]. Taken together, the genome-wide studies suggest that genetic factors for specific IgE responses cannot be attributed to the effect of a single major gene. Specific IgE responsiveness to complex allergens is most likely controlled by *HLA-D* genes with a strong influence of both non-HLA loci and environmental factors.

HLA-region associated generalized immune hyperresponsiveness

Several studies have suggested that allelic variation of class II molecules may influence the Th1- or Th2-like phenotype [39, 40], implying that particular HLA:peptide combinations may favor a strong Th2 response, which in turn results in an exaggerated overall IgE responsiveness. Sib-pair analysis of specific IgE responses to mite in 18 families and a case-control study of 161 non-related individuals revealed a significant difference from expected values in haplotypes shared by affected sibs without any association of particular HLA alleles in a case-control study [41]. HLA class II DR4 and/or DR7 alleles were present in 42.6% of the atopic patients and in only 2.4% of the healthy subjects within a geographic area wherein birch pollen represents the most prominent cause of airborne allergic diseases [42]. Although these results suggest that some particular HLA-class II allele is responsible for the development of allergy to HDM or pollen allergens, we must consider the possibility that susceptibility may be related more to generalized hyperresponsiveness than to specific responses to allergens and that certain alleles of loci within the *HLA* region might be involved in the development of allergic responses to common inhaled allergens.

Marsh et al. postulated the existence of an HLA-associated hyperresponsive state controlled by an additional genetic factor responsible for the overall expression of immune response [43]. This region contains a large number of non-*HLA* genes, many of which are duplicated and polymorphic. A series of genes that is involved in exaggerated immune responses or inflammation has recently been recognized in a chromosome 6p21. They include genes encoding tumor necrosis factor (TNF), transporter antigen peptide (TAP), and PAF acetylhydrolase (PAFAH), which have been implicated in the pathogenesis of either atopy or asthma [44–46]. The proinflammatory cytokine, TNF, shows a constitutional variation in its level of secretion, which is linked to polymorphisms within the *TNF* gene complex. TAP-1 and TAP-2 are also polymorphic genes involved in antigen-processing and presentation. Two mutations in *PAFAH* (Ile198Thr and Ala379Val) likely prolong the activities of PAF, which is involved in several inflammatory processes including allergy. Members of one such gene family also include *PERB11.1* and *PERB11.2*, both of which are encoded in the region between *TNF* and *HLA-B*. The frequency of the PERB11.1*06 allele is 44% in type I psoriasis but only 7% in controls (Pc = 0.003). The major determinant of this association is a single-nucleotide polymorphism (SNP) within intron 4 [47, 48].

Evidence of a linkage between Der p 1-specific IgE antibodies and markers on chromosome 6p21 (*HLA-D* region) was demonstrated in a genome-wide screening within Caucasian families [37]. Exposure to a broad array of different Der p polypeptides renders it difficult to define the genetic contribution of *HLA-D* genes to the expression of Der p-specific IgE responsiveness. Thus, to clarify the genetic contribution of *HLA-D* regions, specific IgE antibodies toward different *Dermatophagoides pteronyssinus* (Der p) polypeptides were detected by immunoblotting analysis, and the transmission/disequilibrium test (TDT) was performed between specific IgE responsiveness toward each different Der p polypeptide and markers on chromosome 6p21 [49]. The study included 299 individuals in 45 Caucasian families participating in the collaborative study on the genetics of asthma (CSGA). Serum samples from 137 individuals who showed elevated specific IgE antibodies toward the Der p crude allergen (> –0.5 log IU/mL) were subjected to immunoblotting analysis. TDT was conducted between the presence of specific IgE antibodies toward each of 12 different Der p polypeptides and 4 polymorphic markers on chromosome 6p21. Although there are, at present, 10 different Der p allergens purified and characterized [50], detailed information on the amino-acid sequence and protein structure of certain Der p polypeptides is currently not available. However, immunoblotting and crossed radio immunoelectrophoresis have identified many other IgE-binding components [51], and immunoblotting analysis has enabled us to identify the overall IgE responsiveness toward the Der p allergens as well as the presence of specific IgE Abs to a panel of the constituent polypeptides. The 196-bp allele of *D6S1281* and the 104-bp allele of *DQCAR* showed significantly increased transmission to specific IgE responders toward a particular Der p polypeptide (120 kD, 55 kD, 45 kD, or 37 kD). In contrast, the 200-bp allele of *D6S1281* and the 204-bp allele of D6S291 showed significantly decreased transmission to specific IgE responders toward a particular Der p polypeptide (120 kD, 90 kD, 52 kD, or 45 kD). These findings supported those of our previous study whereby genes on chromosome 6p21 (*HLA-D* region) may influence the expression of Der p-specific IgE responsiveness in this Caucasian population. Four alleles (196bp and 200bp of *D6S1281*, 104bp of *DQCAR*, and 204bp of *D6S291*) identified in the study [49] could, however, be in tight linkage disequilibrium with a particular allele of *TNF*, *TAP*, *PAFAH*, or *PERB11* genes that may be involved in the amplification of Der p-specific immune responses.

Genes encoding the T-cell receptors (TCRs)

Cognate interaction between TCRs and MHC class II molecules plays an important role in initiating the allergen-specific immune response. TCR is composed of α and β chains in 95% of T cells, and the antigen specificity of the T cell appears to be determined by the arrangement of TCR elements on the α and β chains. Genetic and environmental factors contribute to TCR gene expression and to the development of a specific T-cell response [52]. After ragweed allergen challenge, the clonality of T cells was estimated by analyzing the diversity of TCR V-(D)-J junctional region nucleotide lengths associated with each V alpha and V beta gene family [53]. DNA sequencing of V beta 21 junctional regions in CD8+ T cells revealed a change from polyclonal to oligoclonal expression.

Examination of the TCR V alpha genes of several Lolium perenne I (Lol p I)-specific human T-cell clones also indicated that these cloned cells utilized distinct J alpha genes and that 9 out of 10 clones possessed the V alpha 13 gene [54]. Another study analyzed the expression of 23 V beta and 3 V alpha elements in 56 atopic and nonatopic (NA) individuals from two extended and four nuclear families [55]. The blood samples of symptomatic birch pollen-sensitized individuals that were taken ≤ 6 weeks after the birch pollen season (n = 8) showed a significantly higher frequency of V beta 16.1+ and V beta 20.1+ T cells compared with the blood samples of birch pollen-sensitized individuals that were obtained out of allergen season (n = 10) or from NA individuals ($p < 0.0005$ and $p < 0.0001$, respectively). The distribution of V beta 16.1+ and V beta 20.1+ T cells normalized after the pollen season. The frequency of these V beta-expressing T cells correlated with the levels of allergen-specific IgE Abs. In addition, cat-sensitized individuals (n = 8) showed a significantly higher frequency of V beta 17.1-expressing T cells than did NA individuals ($p < 0.005$). Taken together, these studies demonstrate restricted TCR-V gene usage in specific IgE responses and indicate that this particular usage of TCR V genes may induce Th2 cells and enhance IgE production. The possibility remains that alterations in the T-cell receptor repertoire caused by genetic polymorphism and interactions with the environment could be causal factors in the allergic response.

Two genetic studies have found evidence of linkage between specific IgE responsiveness and *TCRA* and *TCRB*, respectively. In a Japanese population, affected sib-pair (ASP) analyses have provided evidence for linkage both of IgE and asthmatic phenotypes with *TCRB* and nearby markers (*D7S684*) on chromosome 7q35, but no evidence was detected with *TCRA* on chromosome 14q11 [56]. In contrast, Moffatt et al. found a significant linkage to *TCRA* with specific IgE reactions to highly purified major allergens in a study of two independent sets of families, one in the UK and one in Australia [57]. Subsequently, they showed a strong allelic association between a VA8.1 polymorphism (VA8.1(*)2) and reactivity to Der p 2. Reactivity to Der p 2 was confined to subjects who were positive for VA8.1(*)2 and HLA-DRB1(*)1501, demonstrating germline *HLA-DR* and *TCRA* interaction in restricting the response to exogenous antigen [58]. This finding is in line with those of a previous study that demonstrated that *HLA* genes could profoundly influence the TCR V alpha and beta repertoire [59]. Linkage between the *TCR A/D* locus and specific allergic responses was confirmed in a study of 15 extended and 45 nuclear asthmatic families using a panel of 14 microsatellite markers [60]. The *TCRD* locus also remains a candidate for this linkage with chromosome 14q11.2. The biologic role and repertoire of cells bearing the $\gamma\delta$ T-cell receptor has not been fully defined. Indirect evidence, however, implicates $\gamma\delta$ T cells in the cross-regulation of CD4 $\alpha\beta$ T-cell responses. Adoptive transfer of small numbers of $\gamma\delta$ T cells from OVA-tolerant mice selectively suppressed Th2-dependent IgE antibody production without affecting parallel IgG responses [61]. Specific antigen challenge of these $\gamma\delta$ T cells *in vitro* resulted in the production of high levels of γ interferon, which may represent a potential mechanism for the inhibition of Th2 cell proliferation, resulting in suppression of IgE production [62].

Non-HLA, non-TCRs genes

One of the confounding factors for detecting linkage between Der p-specific IgE responsiveness and the *HLA-D* region is the contribution of several non-*HLA* genes to the expression of high IgE responsiveness to complex allergens [5, 10]. Genetic regulation of total IgE levels emerges as a strong determinant of specific IgE responses toward complex allergens. Recently, evidence of a linkage to total IgE levels and/or specific IgE Ab levels has been reported in several chromosomal regions, including chromosome 5q23-q33 [63–65], chromosome 11q13 [66–68], chromosome 12q15-q24.1 [69, 70], and chromosome 13q [68, 71]. Several genes on these chromosome regions, which are not linked to *HLA*, possibly exert their effect on the development of specific IgE responses by amplifying specific IgE responses.

The chromosomal regions 5q31-q33 and 11q13 have been the most extensively studied and thus are relatively well characterized. The candidate gene on chromosome 11q13 encodes the β subunit of the high-affinity IgE receptor (FcϵRI-β), while on chromosome 5q23-q33 a cluster of tightly linked genes is present that includes genes encoding IL-3, IL-4, IL-5, IL-9, IL-13, and GM-CSF. These cytokines play important roles in IgE isotype switching, eosinophil survival, and mast-cell proliferation. The production of IL-4 by PBMCs on stimulation with HDM was significantly higher in children with bronchial asthma than in nonatopic control subjects [72]. Also, IL-4 production showed a close positive correlation with HDM IgE RAST, suggesting that IL-4 is the most important cytokine in upregulation of *in vivo* IgE synthesis against HDM.

Two groups originally reported evidence of a linkage between markers on chromosome 5q31-q33 and total serum IgE levels [63, 64]. Sib-pair analysis of 170 individuals from 11 Amish families revealed evidence of linkage for 5 markers in chromosome 5q31.1 with a gene-controlling total serum IgE concentration. Analysis of total IgE within a subset of 128 IgE antibody-negative sib pairs confirmed the linkage to 5q31.1, especially to the interleukin-4 gene (*IL4*). These findings suggest that *IL4* or a nearby gene in 5q31.1 regulates IgE production in a nonantigen-specific (noncognate) fashion. Two polymorphisms in the IL-4 gene promoter region are associated with elevated levels of total serum IgE [73, 74].

On chromosome 11q13, FcεRI-β is an attractive candidate gene responsible for amplifying specific IgE immune responses, given that FcεRI controls the activation of mast cells and basophils and participates in IgE-mediated antigen presentation. Receptor aggregations by multivalent antigens induce the secretion of allergic mediaters and cytokine gene transcription, such as IL-4, IL-6, TNFα, and GM-CSF. Three coding variants, I181L/V183L, I181L, and E237G, in the *FCER1B* gene have been described previously. An isoleucine to leucine substitution at position 181 (I181L) of FcεRI-β is associated with atopy through maternal descent in a British population [75]. In addition, a glutamic acid-to-glycine substitution (E237G) occurs in approximately 5% of Australian and British populations and is associated with a higher prevalence of atopy and bronchial hyperresponsiveness [76]. Recently, a common −109C/T polymorphism at the promoter region of *FCER1B* was identified [77], and a homozygote of the −109T allele was significantly associated with increased serum total IgE levels in 226 subjects with bronchial asthma ($p = 0.0015$). The strongest evidence for an association ($p = 0.00015$) was obtained when age at onset of asthma was incorporated into the analysis. These regions on chromosome 5q31-q33 and 11q13 are also linked to or associated with parasitic infection [78, 79], supporting the assertion that genes on these regions likely regulate IgE-mediated overall immune responses.

A genome-wide search for genes influencing *Dermatophagoides pteronyssinus* (Der p)-specific IgE responsiveness also provided some evidence in favor of linkage with chromosomes 5q31-q33 and 11q13 in African American families ascertained through an asthmatic sib pair [37]. To clarify the relative contribution of genes on chromosomes 5q31-q33 and 11q13 to specific IgE responsiveness in this African American population, we extended our analysis to IgE responsiveness to a panel of common allergens consisting of *Dermatophagoides farinae* (Der f), *Felis domesticus* (cat), *Canis familiaris* (dog), *Periplaneta americana* (American cockroach), *Lolium perenne* (rye grass), and *Cynodon dactylon* (Bermuda grass) [80]. Specific IgE responses to American cockroach showed evidence of a linkage to chromosomes 5q31-q33 (NPL = 1.23; P = 0.0050) and 11q13 (NPL = 0.96; P = 0.017). Specific IgE responses to dog showed evidence of a linkage with chromosome 5q31-q33 (NPL = 1.15; P = 0.0043). Evidence of a linkage with chromosome 11q13 was also obtained for specific IgE responses to *Dermatophagoides farinae* (NPL = 0.9; P = 0.012), cat (NPL = 0.97; P = 0.035), and Bermuda grass (NPL = 1.16; P = 0.017). The presence of a positive ST response for at least 1 of 30 common allergens showed evidence of a linkage to chromosomes 5q31-q33 (NPL = 1.95; P = 0.017) and 11q13 (NPL = 3.61; P = 0.00058). These data suggest that genes on both chromosomes 5q31-q33 and 11q13 confer susceptibility to upregulated IgE-mediated immune responses in this African American population. The putative genes on chromosomes 5q31-q33 and 11q13, however, had contrasting effects on atopy, which may result from a strong gene-environmental interaction. A multipoint linkage analysis using Haseman-Elston sib-pair methods also provided evidence of a significant linkage between the markers on chromosome 5q and 11q and specific serum IgE levels to HDM and mixed grass in 121 Australian Caucasian nuclear families [81].

Conclusions

Studies of specific IgE immune responsiveness have provided an excellent model to further our understanding of the complex molecular genetics of human immune responsiveness [5]. Much of the interest in genetic control of the immune response to specific allergens has focused on the genes encoding the HLA class II complex and the genes encoding the T-cell receptor, mainly because they are central to the recognition of common environmental allergens. However, it has also been recognized that an appropriate genetic regulation of IgE immune responses to complex allergens requires antigen-nonspecific control [5]. This contention was recently supported by two independent genome-wide linkage analyses, which identified several non-*HLA* regions responsible for the development of specific IgE responsiveness [37, 38]. The actual contribution of these genetic components, including the relative importance of specific *versus* overall IgE regulation, remains obscure, and increasing evidence indicates a role for genetic heterogeneity and complex interactions between genetic and environmental components in the regulation of specific IgE responsiveness. Further studies will examine the presence of variants in a series of candidate genes with an emphasis on their functional outcomes to assess the complex gene-gene and gene-environment interactions.

Acknowledgements

The author thanks the many collaborators who have been involved in the research cited in this chapter, especially David G. Marsh*, Shau-Ku Huang, Kathleen C. Barnes, Linda R. Freidhoff and Eva Ehrlich (Johns Hopkins University School of Medicine, Baltimore, MD, USA); Terri H. Beaty (Johns Hopkins University, School of Hygiene and Public Health, Baltimore, MD, USA); Etsuro Yamaguchi and Yoshikazu Kawakami (Hokkaido University School of Medicine, Sapporo, Japan); and other members of the collaborative study on the genetics of asthma (CSGA).

*Professor David G. Marsh passed away on March 29, 1998.

References

1   Sears MR, Herbison GP, Holdaway MD, Hewitt CJ, Flannery EM, Silva PA (1989) The relative risks of sensitivity to grass pollen, house dust mite and cat dander in the development of childhood asthma. *Clin Exp Allergy* 19: 419–424

2   Hamelmann E, Oshiba A, Schwarze J, Bradley K, Loader J, Larsen GL, Gelfand EW (1997) Allergen-specific IgE and IL-5 are essential for the development of airway hyper-responsiveness. *Am J Respir Cell Mol Biol* 16 (6): 674–682

3   Duffy DL, Mitchell CA, Martin NG (1998) Genetic and environmental risk factors for asthma: a cotwin-control study. *Am J Respir Crit Care Med* 157: 840–845

4   Rosenstreich DL, Eggleston P, Kattan M, Baker D, Slavin RG, Gergen P, Mitchell H, McNiff-Mortimer K, Lynn H, Ownby D, Malveaux F (1997) The role of cockroach allergy and exposure to cockroach allergen in causing morbidity among inner-city children with asthma. *N Engl J Med* 336: 1356–1363

5   Marsh DG, Meyers DA, Bias WB (1981) The epidemiology and genetics of atopic allergy. *N Engl J Med* 305 (26): 1551–1559

6   Sporik R, Holgate ST, Platts-Mills TA, Cogswell JJ (1990) Exposure to house-dust mite allergen (Der p I) and the development of asthma in childhood. A prospective study. *N Engl J Med* 323 (8): 502–507

7   Dizier MH, James A, Faux J, Moffatt MF, Musk AW, Cookson W, Demenais F (1999) Segregation analysis of the specific response to allergens: a recessive major gene controls the specific IgE response to Timothy grass pollen. *Genet Epidemiol* 16 (3): 305–315

8   Marsh DG, Blumenthal MN (1990) Immunogenetics of specific immune responses to allergens in twins and families. In: DG Marsh, MN Blumenthal (eds): *Genetic and environmental factors in clinical allergy*. University of Minnesota Press, Minneapolis, 132–142

9   Newman Taylor AJ, Cullinan P, Lympany PA, Harris JM, Dowdeswell RJ, du Bois RM (1999) Interaction of HLA phenotype and exposure intensity in sensitization to complex platinum salts. *Am J Respir Crit Care Med* 160 (2): 435–438

10 Young RP, Hart BJ, Merrett TG, Read AF, Hopkin JM (1992) House dust mite sensitivity: interaction of genetics and allergen dosage. *Clin Exp Allergy* 22: 205–211

11 Constant S, Pfeiffer C, Woodard A, Pasqualini T, Bottomly K (1995) Extent of T cell receptor ligation can determine the functional differentiation of naive CD4$^+$ T cells. *J Exp Med* 182 (5): 1591–1596

12 Steerenberg PA, Dormans JA, van Doorn CC, Middendorp S, Vos JG, van Loveren H (1999) A pollen model in the rat for testing adjuvant activity of air pollution components. *Inhal Toxicol* 11 (12): 1109–1122

13 Blumenthal MN, Amos BD (1987) Genetic and immunologic basis of atopic responses. *Chest* 91: 176S–184S

14 Chapoval SP, Nabozny GH, Marietta EV, Raymond EL, Krco CJ, Andrews AG, David CS (1999) Short ragweed allergen induces eosinophilic lung disease in HLA-DQ transgenic mice. *J Clin Invest* 12: 1707–1717

15 Freidhoff LR, Ehrlich-Kautzsky E, Meyers DA, Ansari AA, Bias WB, Marsh DG (1988) Association of HLA-DR3 with human immune response to Lol p I and Lol p II allergens in allergic subjects. *Tissue Antigens* 31: 211–219

16 Cardaba B, Vilches C, Martin E, de Andres B, del Pozo V, Hernandez D, Gallardo S, Fernandez JC, Villalba M, Rodriguez R et al (1993) DR7 and DQ2 are positively associated with immunoglobulin-E response to the main antigen of olive pollen (Ole e I) in allergic patients. *Hum Immunol* 38: 293–299

17 Fischer GF, Pickl WF, Fae I, Ebner C, Ferreira F, Breiteneder H, Vikoukal E, Scheiner O, Kraft D (1992) Association between IgE response against Bet v I, the major allergen of birch pollen, and HLA-DRB alleles. *Hum Immunol* 25: 59–71

18 Marsh DG, Hsu SH, Roebber M, Kautzky EE, Freidhoff LR, Meyers DA, Pollard MK, Bias WB (1982) HLA-Dw2: a genetic marker for human immune response to short ragweed pollen allergen Ra5. I. Response resulting primarily from natural antigenic exposure. *J Exp Med* 155: 1439–1451

19 Young RP, Dekker JW, Wordsworth BP, Schou C, Pile KD, Matthiesen F, Rosenberg WM, Bell JI, Hopkin JM, Cookson WO (1994) HLA-DR and HLA-DP genotypes and immunogloblin E responses to common major allergens. *Clin Exp Allergy* 24: 431–439

20 Marsh DG, Meyers DA, Freidhoff LR, Ehrlich-Kautzky E, Roebber M, Norman PS, Hsu SH, Bias WB (1982) HLA-Dw2: a genetic marker for human response to short ragweed pollen allergen Ra 5. II. Response after ragweed immunotherapy. *J Exp Med* 155: 1452–1463

21 Zwollo P, Ehrlich-Kautzky E, Ansari AA, Scarf SJ, Erlich HA, Marsh DG (1991) Molecular studies of human immune response genes for the short ragweed allergen, *Amb a* V. Sequencing of HLA-D second exons in responders and non-responders. *Immunogenetics* 33: 141–151

22 Huang SK, Zwollo P, Marsh DG (1991) Class II MHC restriction of human T-cell responses to short ragweed allergen, *Amb a* V. *Eur J Immunol* 21: 1469–1473

23 Yssel H, Johnson KE, Schneider PV, Wideman J, Terr A, Kastelein R, De Vries JE (1992) T cell activation-inducing epitopes of the house dust mite allergen Der p I-proliferation and lymphokine production patterns by Der p I-specific CD4$^+$ T cell clones. *J Immunol* 148: 738–745

24   Joost van Neerven RJ, Wim van t'Hof, Ringrose JH, Jansen HM, Aalberse RC, Wierenga EA, Kapsenberg ML (1993) T cell epitopes of house dust mite major allergen Der p II. *J Immunol* 151: 2326–2335

25   O'Hehir RE, Eckels DD, Frew AJ, Kay AB, Lamb JR (1988) MHC class II restriction specificity of cloned human T lymphocytes reactive with *Dermatophagoides farinae* (house dust mite). *Immunology* 64: 627–631

26   Marsh DG, Goodfriend L, Bias WB (1977) Basal serum IgE levels and HLA antigens frequencies in allergic subjects. I. Studies with ragweed allergen Ra3. *Immunogenetics* 5: 217

27   A Verhoef, JA Higgins, Thorpe CJ, Marsh SG, Hayball JD, Lamb JR, O'Hehir RE (1993) Clonal analysis of the atopic immune response to the group 2 allergen of Dermatophagoides spp: identification of HLA-DR and –DQ restricted T cell epitopes. *Int Immunol* 5 (12): 1589–1597

28   Brewer JP, Kisselgof AB, Martin TR (1999) Genetic variability in pulmonary physiological, cellular, and antibody responses to antigen in mice. *Am J Respir Crit Care Med* 160 (4): 1150–1156

29   Vaz NM, Levine BB (1970) Immune responses of inbred mice to repeated low doses of antigen: relationship to histocompatibility (H-2) type. *Science* 168 (933): 852–854

30   Dandeu JP, Rabillon J, Perronet R, David B (1992) H2 genotype and IgE immune response to Fel dI, the cat major allergen, in mice. *Immunol Lett* 33 (3): 229–232

31   Mouton D, Prouvost-Danon A, Bouthillier Y, Mevel JC, Abadie A (1980) Variations in the phenotypic expression of an H-2-linked gene contributing to the control of IgE and haemagglutinating antibody responses to ovalbumin. *Ann Immunol (Paris)* 131D (2): 205–215

32   Biozzi G, Mouton D, Sant'Anna OA, Passos HC, Gennari M, Reis MH, Ferreira VC, Heumann AM, Bouthillier Y, Ibanez OM et al (1979) Genetics of immunoresponsiveness to natural antigens in the mouse. *Curr Top Microbiol Immunol* 85: 31–98

33   Marsh DG, Chase GA, Freidhoff LR, Meyers DA, Bias WB (1979) Association of HLA antigens and total serum immunoglobulin E level with allergic response and failure to respond ragweed allergen Ra3. *Proc Nat Acad Sci USA* 76: 2903

34   Ansari AA, Freidhoff LR, Meyers DA, Bias WB, Marsh DG (1989) Human immune responsiveness to Lolium Perenne pollen allergen Lol p III (Rye III) is associated with HLA-DR3 and DR5. *Hum Immunol* 25: 59–71

35   Tovey ER, Sluyter R, Duffy DL, Britton WJ (1998) Immunoblotting analysis of twin sera provides evidence for limited genetic control of specific IgE to house dust mite allergens. *J Allergy Clin Immunol* 101: 491–497

36   Marsh DG, Bias WB, Ishizaka K (1974) Genetic control of basal serum immunoglobulin E level and its effect on specific reagenic sensitivity. *Proc Nat Acad Sci USA* 71: 3588–3592

37   Hizawa N, Freidhoff LR, Chiu YF, Ehrlich E, Luehr CA, Anderson JL, Duffy DL, Dunston GM, Weber JL, Huang SK et al (1998) Genetic regulation of *Dermatophagoides pteronyssinus*-specific IgE responsiveness: a genome-wide multipoint linkage analysis in

families recruited through 2 asthmatic sibs. Collaborative Study on the Genetics of Asthma (CSGA). *J Allergy Clin Immunol* 102 (3): 436–442

38 Wjst M (1999) Specific IgE – one gene fits all? German Asthma Genetics Group. *Clin Exp Allergy* 29 (Suppl 4): 5–10

39 Murray JS, Madri J, Tite J, Carding SR, Bottomly K (1989) MHC control of CD4[+] T cell subset activation. *J Exp Med* 170: 2135

40 Schountz T, Kasselman JP, Martinson FA, Brown L, Murray JS (1996) MHC genotype controls the capacity of ligand density to switch T helper (Th)-1/Th-2 priming *in vivo*. *J Immunol* 157: 3893–3901

41 Torres-Galvan MJ, Quiralte J, Blanco C, Castillo R, Carrillo T, Perez-Aciego P, Sanchez-Garcia F (1999) Linkage of house dust mite allergy with the HLA region. *Ann Allergy Asthma Immunol* 82 (2): 198–203

42 Senechal H, Geny S, Desvaux FX, Busson M, Mayer C, Aron Y, Oster JP, Bessot JC, Peltre G, Pauli G et al (1999) Genetics and specific immune response in allergy to birch pollen and food: evidence of a strong, positive association between atopy and the HLA class II allele HLA-DR7. *J Allergy Clin Immunol* 104: 395–401

43 Marsh DG, Hsu SH, Hussain R, Meyers DA, Freidhoff LR, Bias WB (1980) Genetics of human immune response to allergens. *J Allergy Clin Immunol* 65 (5): 322–332

44 Moffatt MF, Cookson WOCM (1997) Tumour necrosis factor haplotypes and asthma. *Hum Mol Genet* 6: 551–554

45 Ismail A, Bousaffara R, Kaziz J, Zili J, el Kamel A, Tahar Sfar M, Remadi S, Chouchane L (1997) Polymorphism in transporter antigen peptides gene (TAP1) associated with atopy in Tunisians. *J Allergy Clin Immunol* 99: 216–223

46 Kruse S, Mao XQ, Heinzmann A, Blattmann S, Roberts MH, Braun S, Gao PS, Forster J, Kuehr J, Hopkin JM et al (2000) The Ile198Thr and Ala379Val variants of plasmatic Paf-Acetylhydrolase impair catalytical activities and are associated with atopy and asthma. *Am J Hum Genet* 66 (5): 1522–1530

47 Allen MH, Veal C, Faassen A, Powis SH, Vaughan RW, Trembath RC, Barker JN (1999) A non-HLA gene within the MHC in psoriasis. *Lancet* 8: 353 (9164): 1589–1590

48 Tay GK, Hui J, Gaudieri S, Schmitt-Egenolf M, Martinez OP, Leelayuwat C, Williamson JF, Eiermann TH, Dawkins RL (2000) PERB11 (MIC): a polymorphic MHC gene is expressed in skin and single nucleotide polymorphisms are associated with psoriasis. *Clin Exp Immunol* 119 (3): 553–558

49 Hizawa N, Collins G, Rafnar T, Huang SK, Duffy DL, Weber JL, Freidhoff LR, Ehrlich E, Marsh DG, Beaty TH et al (1998) Linkage analysis of *Dermatophagoides pteronyssinus*-specific IgE responsiveness with polymorphic markers on chromosome 6p21 (HLA-D region) in Caucasian families by the transmission/disequilibrium test. Collaborative Study on the Genetics of Asthma (CSGA) *J Allergy Clin Immunol* 102(3): 443–448

50 King TP, Hoffman D, Lowenstein H, Marsh DG, Platts-Mills TAE, Thomas W (1995) Allergen Nomenclature. J Allergy Clin Immunol 96: 5–14

51 Shibasaki M, Isoyama S, Takita H (1994) Influence of age on IgE responsiveness to

Dermatophagoides farinae: an immunoblot study. *Int Arch Allergy Immunol* 103: 53–58

52 Silver J, Gulwani-Akolkar B, Akolkar PN (1995) The influence of genetics, environment, and disease state on the human T-cell receptor repertoire. *Ann NY Acad Sci* 756: 28–52

53 Yurovsky VV, Weersink EJ, Meltzer SS, Moore WC, Postma DS, Bleecker ER, White B (1998) T-Cell repertoire in the blood and lungs of atopic asthmatics before and after ragweed challenge. *Am J Respir Cell Mol Biol* 18 (3): 370–383

54 Mohapatra SS, Mohapatra S, Yang M, Ansari AA, Parronchi P, Maggi E, Romagnani S (1994) Molecular basis of cross-reactivity among allergen-specific human T cells: T-cell receptor V alpha gene usage and epitope structure. *Imunology* 81 (1): 15–20

55 Beyer K, Hausler T, Kircher M, Nickel R, Wahn U, Renz H (1999) Specific V beta T cell subsets are associated with cat and birch pollen allergy in humans. *J Immunol* 162 (2): 1186–1191

56 Noguchi E, Shibasaki M, Arinami T, Takeda K, Kobayashi K, Matsui A, Hamaguchi H (1998) Evidence for linkage between the development of asthma in childhood and the T-cell receptor beta chain gene in Japanese. *Genomics* 47 (1): 121–124

57 Moffatt MF, Hill MR, Cornelis F, Schou C, Faux JA, Young RP, James AL, Ryan G, le Souef P, Musk AW et al (1994) Genetic linkage of T-cell receptor alpha/delta complex to specific IgE responses. *Lancet* 343 (8913): 1597–1600

58 Moffatt MF, Schou C, Faux JA, Cookson WO (1997) Germline TCR-A restriction of immunoglobulin E responses to allergen. *Immunogenetics* 46 (3): 226–230

59 Gulwani-Akolkar B, Shi B, Akolkar PN, Ito K, Bias WB, Silver J (1995) Do HLA genes play a prominent role in determining T cell receptor V alpha segment usage in humans? *J Immunol* 154(8): 3843–3851

60 Mansur AH, Bishop DT, Markham AF, Morton NE, Holgate ST, Morrison JF (1999) Suggestive evidence for genetic linkage between IgE phenotypes and chromosome 14q markers. *Am J Respir Crit Care Med* 159 (6): 1796–1802

61 McMenamin C, Pimm C, McKersey M, Holt PG (1994) Regulation of IgE responses to inhaled antigen in mice by antigen-specific gamma delta T cells. *Science* 265 (5180): 1869–1871

62 McMenamin C, McKersey M, Kuhnlein P, Hunig T, Holt PG (1995) Gamma delta T cells down-regulate primary IgE responses in rats to inhaled soluble protein antigens. *J Immunol* 154 (9): 4390–4394

63 Marsh DG, Neely JD, Breazeale DR, Ghosh B, Freidhoff LR, Ehrlich E, Schou C, Krishnaswamy G, Beaty TH (1994) Linkage analysis of IL4 and other chromosome 5q31.1 markers and total serum immunoglobulin E concentrations. *Science* 264: 1152–1156

64 Meyers DA, Postma DS, Panhuysen CIM, Xu J, Amelung PJ, Levitt RC, Bleecker ER (1994) Evidence for a locus regulating total serum IgE levels mapping to chromosome 5. *Genomics* 23: 464–470

65 Collaborative Study on the Genetics of Asthma (1997) A genome-wide search for asthma susceptibility loci in ethnically diverse population. *Nature Genet* 15: 389–392

66   Cookson WOCM, Sharp PA, Faux JA, Hopkin JM (1989) Linkage between immuno-globulin E response underlying asthma and rhinitis and chromosome 11q. *Lancet* i: 1292–1295

67   Sandford AJ, Shirakawa T, Moffat MF, Daniels SE, Ra C, Faux JA, Young RP, Naka-mura Y, Lathrop GM, Cookson WO et al (1993) Localisation of atopy and the β sub-unit of high affinity IgE receptor (FcεRI) on chromosome 11q. *Lancet* 341: 332–334

68   Daniels SE, Bhattacharrya S, James A, Leaves NI, Young A, Hills MR, Faux JA, Ryan GF, le Souef PN, Lathrop GM et al (1996) A genome wide search for quantitative trait loci underlying asthma. *Nature* 383: 247–250

69   Barnes KC, Neely JD, Duffy DL, Freidhoff LR, Breazeale DR, Schou C, Naidu RP, Lev-ett PN, Renault B, Kucherlapati R et al (1996) Linkage of asthma and total serum IgE concentration to markers on chromosome 12q: Evidence from Afro-Caribbean and Caucasian populations. *Genomics* 37: 41–50

70   Nickel R, Wahn U, Hizawa N, Maestri N, Duffy DL, Barnes KC, Beyer K, Forster J, Bergmann R, Zepp F et al (1997) Evidence of linkage of chromosome 12q15-q24.1 markers to high total serum IgE concentrations in children of the German Multicenter Allergy Study. *Genomics* 46: 159–162

71   Kimura K, Noguchi E, Shibasaki M, Arinami T, Yokouchi Y, Takeda K, Yamakawa-Kobayashi K, Matsui A, Hamaguchi H (1999) Linkage and association of atopic asth-ma to markers on chromosome 13 in the Japanese population. *Hum Mol Genet* 8 (8): 1487–1490

72   Kimura M, Tsuruta S, Yoshida T (2000) IL-4 production by PBMCs on stimulation with mite allergen is correlated with the level of serum IgE antibody against mite in children with bronchial asthma. *J Allergy Clin Immunol* 105 (2 Pt 1): 327–332

73   Rosenwasser LJ, Klemm DJ, Dresback JK, Inamura H, Mascali JJ, Klinnert M, Borish L (1995) Promoter polymorphisms in the chromosome 5 gene cluster in asthma and atopy. *Clin Exp Allergy* 25 (Suppl 2): 74–78

74   Suzuki I, Yamaguchi E, Hizawa N, Itoh A, Kawakami Y (1999) A new polymorphism in the 5' flanking region of the human interleukin (IL)-4 gene. *Immunogenetics* 49 (7–8): 738–739

75   Shirakawa T, Li A, Dubowitz M, Dekker JW, Shaw AE, Faux JA, Ra C, Cookson WO, Hopkin JM (1994) Association between atopy and variants of the beta subunit of the high-affinity immunoglobulin E receptor. Nat Genet 7(2): 125–129

76   Hill MR, Cookson WOCM (1996) A new variant of the β subunit of the high-affinity receptor for immunoglobulin E (FcεRI-β E237G): associations with measures of atopy and bronchial hyper-responsiveness. *Hum Mol Genet* 5: 959–962

77   Hizawa N, Yamaguchi E, Jinushi E, Kawakami Y (2000) A common FCER1B gene pro-moter polymorphism* influences total serum IgE levels in a Japanese population. *Am J Respir Crit Care Med* 161: 906–909

78   Marquet S, Abel L, Hillaire D, Dessein H, Kalil J, Feingold J, Weissenbach J, Dessein AJ (1996) Genetic localization of a locus controlling the intensity of infection by Schisto-soma mansoni on chromosome 5q31-q33. *Nature Genet* 14: 181–184

79   Palmer LJ, Pare PD, Faux JA, Moffatt MF, Daniels SE, LeSouef PN, Bremner PR, Mock-
     ford E, Gracey M, Spargo R et al (1997) FcεR1-β polymorphism and total serum IgE
     levels in endemically parasitized Australian Aborigines. *Am J Hum Genet* 61: 182–188
80   Hizawa N, Freidhoff LR, Ehrlich E, Chiu YF, Duffy DL, Schou C, Dunston GM, Beaty
     TH, Marsh DG, Barnes KC et al (1998) Genetic influences of chromosomes 5q31-q33
     and 11q13 on specific IgE responsiveness to common inhaled allergens among African
     American families. Collaborative Study on the Genetics of Asthma (CSGA). *J Allergy
     Clin Immunol* 102 (3): 449–453
81   Palmer LJ, Daniels SE, Rye PJ, Gibson NA, Tay GK, Cookson WO, Goldblatt J, Burton
     PR, LeSouef PN (1998) Linkage of chromosome 5q and 11q gene markers to asthma-
     associated quantitative traits in Australian children. *Am J Respir Crit Care Med* 158 (6):
     1825–1830

Genetic variation at the HLA and TCR loci and the development of allergy and asthma

Adel H. Mansur

Molecular Medicine Unit, Clinical Sciences Building, St. James's University Hospital, Leeds, LS9 7TF, UK

Background

Antigen-presenting cells (APCs), including B cells, airway dendritic cells, tissue macrophages, and skin Langerhans cells, engulf and process protein antigens into small peptides of approximately 12 to 17 amino acids in length. Processed peptides bind to the binding groove of the major histocompatibility molecules (MHC), forming a peptide-MHC complex that is translocated to the cell surface. The presented peptide is recognised by a specific T cell through its receptor the TCR. T cells also carry other surface molecules, which are important to antigen recognition. These include the TCR-associated CD3 molecule, CD4 molecules on helper T cells (CD4+ T cells), and CD8 on cytotoxic T cells (CD8+ T cells). CD4+ T cell recognises processed peptides of exogenous antigens bound to the MHC class II, while CD8+ T cells generally recognise peptides processed from endogenous antigens (e.g., virally infected cells) that are bound to MHC class I.

Activated CD4+ T cells interact with B cells in a cognate (specific) manner through the TCR-peptide-MHC class II complex or non-cognately (non-specific) through the secretion of cytokines. B cell interaction with T cells leads to B cell activation, which may then develop into an antibody-secreting plasma cell. The antibody class produced by a plasma cell depends on the cytokine profile produced by the CD4+ T cells. There are two types of helper CD4+ T cells (Th) described [1]. Th1 cells express predominantly interleukin-2 (IL-2) and interferon-γ (IFNγ) but not IL-4 or IL-5, while Th2 cells express predominantly IL-4, IL-5, IL-10, and IL-13 but not IL-2 or IFNγ. Both cell types express IL-3 and granulocyte-macrophage colony-stimulating factor (GM-CSF) (Fig. 1). A third cell type (Th0) has also been described that expresses all of the above cytokines. The dominance of Th1 or Th2 cell type in any immune response may determine the type of autoimmune disease encountered [2, 3]. The Th2 subtype secretes a profile of cytokines that is optimally tuned for the stimulation of an allergic response. However, the expression of these cytokines is not exclusive to T cells. It has been shown that mast cells express IL-4 [4 ,5] and IL-4 [6], eosinophils express IL-5 and GM-CSF [7], and epithelial cells express GM-CSF

The Hereditary Basis of Allergic Diseases, edited by Stephen T. Holgate and John W. Holloway

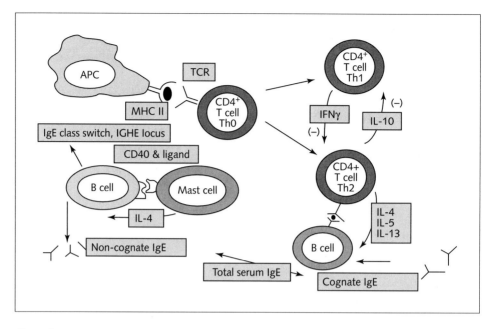

Figure1

Molecular mechanisms in asthma and allergy. Illustration of the central role played by the HLA and TCR antigens in the handling and processing of antigens and initiation of the immune response. Th2 cells play a central role in the propagation of allergic response. IL-4 and IL-13 are the main cytokines involved in immunoglobulin switch to class E chain in B cells, which are antagonised by IFNγ and IL-10.

[8]. IL-4 is crucial for the development and functioning of Th2 cells, including their ability to secrete IL-5, which promotes eosinophil growth, maturation, and survival [9].

In addition to interaction between peptide-MHC complex and TCR, T cell activation requires co-stimulation. One co-stimulatory pathway is mediated through CD28 on the T cell and its counter receptors CD80 (B7-1) and CD86 (B7-2) present on the APC. Interaction between CD28 and either CD80 or CD86 is required for a productive T-cell response in terms of proliferation and cytokine production. Blockade of this interaction in specific circumstances can lead to unresponsiveness of T cells, a phenomenon described as "anergy" [10]. CTLA4, a T cell molecule related to CD28, functions as an inhibitory receptor for CD80 and CD86 [11]. CD28 is constitutively expressed on T cells, and CD86 is present on resting APC, whereas both CTLA4 on T cells and CD80 on APC are upregulated upon activation [12]. Therefore, CD28/CD86 interaction may predominate in activation of resting cells, with CD80 acting on activated APC, and CTLA4 may have a later regulatory role. It has been shown that CD28/CD80/CD86 play a role in Th2 cell activation and in the production of IL-4 and IL-5 [13].

Immunoglobulin (Ig) production occurs in B cell and plasma cells. These molecules are constructed from two heavy chains and two light chains (κ or λ) linked by disulphide bridges and have two functional domains. The heavy chains are encoded by genes, which map to human chromosome 14q32 region; the κ light-chain genes map to 2p12, and the λ light-chain genes map to 22q11. The antigen-binding specificity is determined by the NH2 terminus of the Ig heavy and light chains, which are extremely variable. The COOH terminus of the immunoglobulins' heavy chain determines the effector function of the molecule. The variable (V) regions of both heavy and light chains combine to form the antigen-binding domain. Within the basic framework of the variable domain are hypervariable or complementarity-determining regions 1 through 3 (CDRs), of which CDR3 is directly involved in the interaction with the antigen. The remainder of the molecule, the constant (C) region, varies only between different classes of Ig polypeptide (δ, μ, γ, α, ε heavy chains for IgD, IgM, IgG, IgA, and IgE classes, respectively).

The genetic recombination between the constant and variable regions generates functional genes that are able to encode the heavy chains of antibody molecules. Initially, the μ chain is used to generate the IgM molecules. Subsequently, in the presence of antigens and T cells, immunoglobulin class switch occurs to γ, α, or ε constant chains. The immunoglobulin switch to class E requires at least two signals: one is delivered by a cytokine, IL-4 or IL-13, and the other is a B cell activating signal [14]. IL-4 is necessary, but not sufficient, for the induction of IgE synthesis. Th2 cells are crucial for IgE synthesis both by producing IL-4 and delivering activating signal to B cells through the cognate interaction between the TCR and MHC class II antigens [15]. B cell activating signals also involve the binding of CD40 molecule on the B cell surface to its ligand (CD40L) on the T cell surface [16, 17]. It has also been shown that basophils and mast cells can interact with B cells through the CD40 molecule and its binding ligand and hence may facilitate a switch to IgE isotype in a non-cognate manner [18].

Genetic restriction of the specific allergic response

The ability of TCR to interact with a particular peptide-MHC complex is restricted by polymorphism within the MHC and TCR. This limits the ability of T cells to respond to an antigen, which is a critical step in the regulation of the immune response and involves the discrimination between self and foreign antigens (self-tolerance); if this process breaks down, autoimmune disease results. Inappropriate or misdirected immune response to foreign antigens (e.g., inhaled aeroallergens), on the other hand, results in hypersensitivity or allergy. Given their central role in anti-

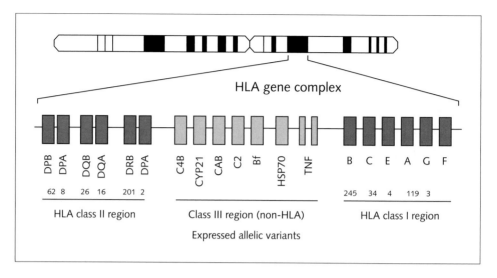

Figure 2
HLA gene complex on chromosome 6p21.3.

gen presentation and recognition, both the MHC and TCR play a pivotal role in the control of the allergic responses.

The major histocompatibility complex (MHC)

The classical MHC or HLA molecules are encoded by highly polymorphic gene families located in about 8 Mb region of the short arm of the chromosome (6p21.3) (Fig. 2). The transcribed molecules are membrane-bound glycoproteins that bind and present processed antigens to the T cells.

The MHC class I A, B, and C molecules are composed of MHC heavy chain (45 kDa), non-covalently associated with a nonpolymorphic polypeptide, β2-microglobulin (12 kDa), which is encoded on chromosome 15. The heavy chain consists of three membrane-external domains (α1, α2, and α3), a transmembrane portion, and a cytoplasmic tail. The polymorphism arising from the various allelic forms of the class I genes mainly localise to α1 and α2 domains. To date, 119 class I A, 245 class I B, and 59 class I C alleles have been described [19]. Structural studies have shown that the polymorphisms are grouped together in and around the peptide-binding site and that they are likely to be of functional significance (Fig. 3). MHC class I antigens are expressed on all nucleated cells (except fetal trophoblast and platelets) [20]. In order for them to present an antigen, it is

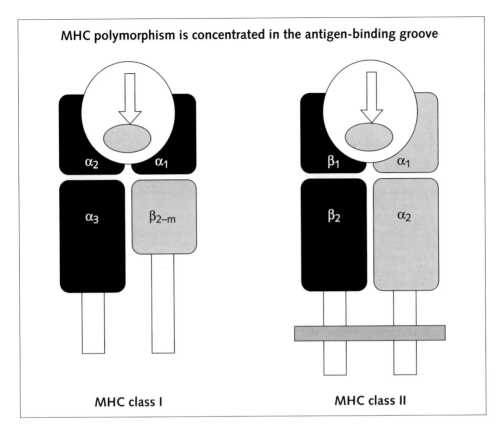

Figure 3
The MHC class I and class II molecules. Abbreviations: β2–m, β2-microglobulin.

necessary for the antigen to be synthesised within the presenting cells [21]. MHC class I antigens play a central role in the recognition of endogenous antigen by CD8+ T cells.

Class II genes are encoded by the HLA-D region of the MHC and are comprised of three main subclasses (DR, DQ, DP). An expressed class II MHC molecule consists of α chain (35 kDa encoded by the A gene, e.g., DRA), which is non-covalently bound to a β chain (28 kDa encoded by the B gene, e.g., DRB). Both A and B genes are located on chromosome 6p and are highly polymorphic [22, 23]. Both chains have two membrane-external domains (α1 and α2, and β1 and β2, respectively), each chain possessing a transmembrane portion and a cytoplasmic tail (Fig. 3). The three principal class II antigens differ in their degree of allelic polymorphism. The extensive polymorphism of class II molecules is confined mainly to the peptide-binding groove of each molecule. Polymorphism in the groove results in a differential ability to bind particular peptides and is the structural basis of MHC restriction of the response to foreign antigens. The tissue distribution of the MHC class II antigens is limited [24]. The main class II types (DR, DP, DQ) are found on B cells, monocytes, macrophages, dendritic cells, and activated T cells.

HLA-DR

The HLA-DR region contains a single DRA gene, but multiple DRB genes. The DRA gene shows limited polymorphism, with only two recognised alleles [22,25]. In contrast, the DRB genes are highly polymorphic. In addition to allelic variation within the DRB genes, more than one DRB gene may be expressed, and the number of DRB loci within the sub-region can also vary. Nine DRB loci have been described, five of which are pseudogenes. Most DR haplotypes express two DRB genes, with only two haplotypes expressing a single gene. The DRB1 gene is present in all haplotypes and is the most polymorphic, with 201 alleles currently described. The second DRB locus (DRB3, DRB4, or DRB5) varies between haplotypes. All three secondary loci exhibit polymorphism, which is more limited than that seen for DRB1 [26].

HLA-DQ

The HLA-DQ region contains four genes grouped into two pairs. DQA1 and DQB1 genes are both expressed, giving rise to a glycoprotein heterodimer. DQA2 and DQB2, however, are unlikely to produce protein products. Both the DQA1 and DQB1 genes are polymorphic, with 16 DQA alleles and 26 DQB alleles currently recognised [26]. In contrast to HLA-DR, the DQ-α chain is very polymorphic and contains a hypervariable loop between residues 48 and 56, which is one of the most polymorphic structures known [27]. However, not all these polymorphisms localise within the antigen-binding groove. Most of the polymorphisms in DQB are within the β_1 domain [28].

HLA-DP

The HLA-DP region also contains four genes grouped into two pairs. DPA2 and DPB2 are non-functional pseudogenes [29], while DPA1 and DPB1 result in an expressed heterodimer. A large number of alleles (62 to date) are found at the DNA level for DPB1, but the resulting amino-acid variation is less than that seen for the DRB and DRQ genes. DPA1 variability is limited, with eight alleles known [26].

Non-classical HLA and non-HLA genes in the MHC class I/II regions

The HLA region also contains a large number of other genes with various functions. In the class I region, there are known to be 17 genes, three of which only (HLA-E, F, and G) are known to be transcribed [30]. The functions of these genes remain to be elucidated, although the HLA-G gene is found to be expressed mainly in fetal cytotrophoblast cells and hence may function as a fetal antigen-presenting and/or antigen-recognition molecule and could be involved in the maternal tolerance of the placenta [31]. Other genes include complement genes, the tumour necrosis factor locus, and genes that encode proteins that function in the transportation of exogenous peptides within the cells (TAP1 and TAP2) [32].

Linkage disequilibrium within the MHC

Because of the close proximity of different MHC classes loci, and because of their high polymorphism, particular combinations of alleles or haplotypes are seen more often than would be expected by chance (linkage disequilibrium) [33]. The strength of linkage disequilibrium between these loci led to the description of different extended haplotypes in different ethnic groups. This phenomenon is particularly important in association studies, in which the detection of an association to one particular allele could be spurious and caused by association to another locus in linkage disequilibrium with that allele. Indeed, the DQ locus lies between the DR and DP loci, and all three are contained within approximately 1 Mb [34].

Linkage/association of the HLA region (6p21.3) to asthma and allergy

Evidence implicating the HLA genes in allergy has been provided by both genome screen and candidate-gene studies. Daniels et al. (1996) reported linkage of eosinophilia to markers close to the MHC class I genes [35]. The Collaborative Study on the Genetics of Asthma (1997) observed linkage of asthma to marker D6S1281, which maps near to the HLA region [36]. In the same population, positive transmission disequilibrium was reported between specific IgE to HDM and markers close to HLA-D [37]. A third genome screen was performed in a founder Hutterites population, which reported an association of asthma and atopy to MHC class II genes. However, no linkage was observed in the latter study, suggesting perhaps only a modest effect for the HLA in this inbred population [38]. Similarly, other studies used the candidate-gene approach and showed either association or linkage with the HLA. Young et al. reported a number of weak associations between DRB1 alleles and IgE responsiveness to specific allergens in 77 nuclear and 7 extended families [39]. In a German population, sib-pair analysis showed linkage of specific IgE to

HDM to HLA-DPB, DRB, and DQB [40]. In contrast, one recent genome screen observed no linkage between HLA markers and HDM sensitisation in a multiethnic white population [41]. The overall evidence leaves little doubt that the HLA genes are linked to and associated with asthma and allergy. However, the magnitude of the relative risk contributed by the HLA remains unknown. The generally modest and sometimes negative linkage with the HLA would suggest perhaps a strong genetic role for non-HLA loci. The relative risk contributed by the HLA genes to the allergic diathesis is likely to vary, however, and would depend on the allergic phenotype studied.

Within the HLA, DRB1 genes are the most polymorphic and therefore are most extensively investigated. DQ and DP genes are less polymorphic but have also been the focus of many studies. Reports of association between various HLA antigens and different allergic entities are listed in Table 1. A large number of these associations remain unconfirmed, and the number of subjects studied generally has not approached that required to establish an unequivocal HLA association. The restriction of the IgE response to ragweed (*Ambrosia artemisifolia*) by HLA was one of the first to be reported [42] and was subsequently confirmed by others [43, 44]. This was refined to the association of a minor ragweed allergen *Amb a* V and HLA-DRB1*1501(DR2)-associated haplotype. HLA-DR2 or DR2-associated genes were also found to be associated with allergic asthma in patients with ragweed atopy [45].

In an international HLA workshop, specific IgE responsiveness to eight highly purified allergens (*Lol p* V, *Amb a* V, *Par o* I, *Bet v* I, *Cry i* I, *Fel d* I, *Alt a* I, and *Der p* I) were examined in 1006 atopic individuals from 13 population groups. The main emphasis was on correlation with polymorphism of the HLA-DRB1 gene [53]. The most consistent association was seen in individuals with DRB1*04 and IgE responsiveness to *Alt a* I. The DRB1*04 association was observed across ethnic and racial lines, while the DRB1*14 association was observed in three Caucasian groups. The association between DRB1*15 and IgE responsiveness to *Amb a* V was confirmed in the U.S. Caucasoid population. Some other associations were also observed in some ethnic groups but were not confirmed in others, including associations of IgE responsiveness to HDM allergens *Der p* I and DRB1*04 (in Swedish Caucasoid) and DRB1*03 (in Italian Caucasoid).

The lack of recognition of the problem of reactivity to multiple allergens by some of the studies listed in Table 1 might have accounted for some of the observed discrepancy. For example, in one pool of approximately 200 subjects there were reports of significant relationships between HLA DR alleles and four antigens (*Amb a* V, *Lol p* I, *Lol p* II, and *Lol p* III) [43, 50, 51, 56]. Including predominant numbers of subjects who demonstrate reactivity to multiple allergens in such studies might confound the dissection of association to individual allergens. The high prevalence of multiple reactivity to allergens in the population makes the recruitment of subjects with specific reactivity to only one allergen difficult. In some cases, association to particular allergen sensitivity may be spurious and related to the general

Table 1 - Published associations between HLA-MHC class II antigens and the allergic diathesis. Data are listed according to the MHC class II numerical order.

HLA antigen/allele	Associated trait	Population (number)	Refs.
Haplotype DRB1*0101, 02,	Non-biting midge allergen (*Chi t* 1)		[46]
DQA1*0101, DQB1*0501	Cockroach allergen	Hutterites African-American (109)	[47]
HLA-DRB3*0101	Birch tree pollen (*Bet v* I)	Australian (37) Danish (41)	[48] [49]
DRB1*03 & DRB1*11	Rye grass antigens (*Lolium perenne*)		[50, 51]
DRB1*03	Acid anhydrides		[52]
DRB1*04	*Alterneria A.* (*Alt a* I.) & HDM (*Der p* I)		[53]
	Alt a I & Cat hair (*Fel d*)	Caucasian (84)	[39]
	Birch pollens, atopy, asthma		[54]
	ABPA		[55]
DR5	Ragweed antigen (*Amb a* VI)		[56]
DRB1*07	Olive pollen allergen (*Ole e* I)		[57, 58]
	Atopy	Caucasian (95)	[59]
	Total IgE	Caucasian (181)	[60]
	Birch pollen, atopy, asthma	Caucasian (84)	[54]
	Nasal polyposis	Caucasian (100)	[61]
	ABPA		[55]
	Citrus red mite & HDM asthma	Korean (189)	[62]
Haplotype DRB1*11, DQA1*0501, DQB1*0301	Asthma	Venezuelan (135)	[63]
DRB1*14	*Alternaria A.* (*Alt a* I.)		[53]
HLA-DRB1*1501	Ragweed allergen (*Amb a* V)		[42–45]
HLA-DRB1*15 &	Asthma	Caucasian (176)	[64]
HLA-DRB1*1501,03	ABPA		[55]
DQB1*0501, 0502 (protective)	Atopy	Caucasian (95)	[59]
	Isocyanate-induced asthma	Italian (94)	[65]
	Red cedar-induced asthma	Caucasian (119)	[66]
DQ2	ABPA		[55]
DQA1*0104 & DQB1*0503	Isocyanate-induced asthma	Italian (94)	[65]
DQB1*06 & DQB1*03	Red cedar-induced asthma	Caucasian (119)	[66]
DQA1*0301	HDM (*Der f*)		[67]
DPB1*0301	Aspirin-induced asthma		[68]
DQw2	Aspirin-induced asthma		[69]

Abbreviations: Alt a *I, the mould* Alternaria alternata; *HDM, house dust mite;* Der p *I,* Dermatophagoides pternyssinus; *Der f,* Dermatophagoides farinae; *Fel d,* Felis domesticus; *ABPA, allergic bronchopulmonary aspergillosis.*

atopic effect. This is best illustrated in the case of the DRB1*07 genotype. This particular allele has been associated by different groups with specific allergy to olive pollen allergen (*Ole e* I) [58], birch tree pollen (*Bet v* I) [54], citrus red mite- and HDM-sensitive asthma [62], allergic bronchopulmonary aspergillosis [55], and nasal polyposis [61]. In addition, it has been strongly associated with the general atopic status (defined as positive skin test reactivity to one or more of the 17 common allergens tested, raised total serum IgE, or BHR) [59]. The latter study showed the presence of the DRB1*04 and DRB1*07 alleles in 39.2% of the patients but in only 2.5% of the controls. DRB1*07 has been strongly associated with total serum IgE [60], atopy and asthma [54], and citrus mite-induced occupational asthma [62]. Collectively, these studies seem to implicate DRB1*07 in predisposition to general atopic status rather than influencing one particular allergic responses. Foreign aeroallergens are proteins with a complex structure and are endocytosed and degraded to small peptides before binding to the MHC groove. Only some peptide residues of this complex seem to extend to the MHC groove [70]. This could explain why sensitisation to many different molecules could be associated with a restricted allele or haplotype, although aeroallergens differ widely in structure. An alternative explanation for this lack of stringent specificity is that a very similar structure in different or related proteins may act as an allergen in various and sometimes unrelated species, thereby reducing the apparently great diversity of allergens. This is consistent with the concept of a pan-allergen that is responsible in some patients for cross-allergic manifestations caused by various or unrelated species of plant or food allergens [71].

The presence of extended-haplotypes and linkage disequilibrium across the HLA region represents a particular confounding factor in the studies of HLA genetics. The finding of positive association with any particular allele may indicate a cause-effect relationship or may be secondary to another allele in linkage disequilibrium with that allele.

Some HLA alleles are likely to adopt a protective role against the predisposition to allergic disease. The strongest evidence for protection is seen with the DQA1*0103, DQB1*0502 haplotype. This haplotype is significantly less prevalent in atopics compared with normal control [59]. DQB1*05 positive subjects display a trend toward low total serum IgE and low incidence of skin test reactivity to common allergens [60]. Protection against isocyanate-induced asthma was proposed by the observation of the lower prevalence of DQA1*0103, DQB1*0502 haplotype in exposed and affected workers as compared with exposed and non-affected workers [65,72,73]. Among workers exposed to the western red cedar, asthma is more prevalent in subjects lacking this haplotype [66].

The role of HLA class I antigens (A, B, and C) in allergic disease remains less clear. There have been some reports of association with either HLA class I antigens or alleles. In particular, HLA-B8 (which is in linkage disequilibrium with DR3) was reported to be associated with atopy [74, 75] and atopic asthma [76]. However, this association was not observed in two studies [77, 78]. It is unclear whether the association between asthma and atopy and HLA class I alleles is causal or due to linkage-disequilibrium to HLA class II alleles or indeed other loci in the region.

In summary, there is adequate evidence to implicate the HLA alleles/antigens in the predisposition to or protection against asthma or allergy. However, the magnitude of this effect remains unknown. It is likely that the HLA role in this context will become more clear when studied in conjunction with other non-HLA loci, in particular the TCR genes.

The T cell receptor (TCR)

The TCR is comprised of either the $\alpha\beta$ form or the $\gamma\delta$ form. The TCR $\alpha\beta$ form is present on 95% of the T cells in peripheral blood. This receptor is non-covalently associated with three other molecules that constitute the CD3 complex [79] and two signal transduction elements, η and ζ. CD3 is involved in TCR assembly and cell surface expression [80,81].

The TCR $\gamma\delta$ is also expressed in association with the CD3 complex [82], and the $\gamma\delta$ T cells constitute between 0.1% and 10% of the peripheral blood T cell population [83, 84]. These T cells are localised in the skin, uterus, tongue, lung, mammary glands, and intestinal epithelia in mice and in the blood and spleen in humans and are found in all vertebrates. The function of the $\gamma\delta$ T cell is not yet fully clear, but it may play a role in immune surveillance [85]; in particular, a protective role against bacterial and parasitic infection has been suggested [86–89]. The localisation of these cells to epithilial surfaces in the body supports this hypothesis. Additionally, these cells may also play an important role in the regulation of IgE production. The presence of $\gamma\delta$ T cells in mucosal surfaces such as lung epithelium, where allergens initiate IgE responses, led to the suggestion of a possible protective role played by these cells in which they selectively suppress IgE production, hence limiting the inflammatory damage [85, 90]. This notion is contradicted by the observation of decreased specific IgE, IgG1, and IL-5 release as well as eosinophil recruitment and T-cell infiltration in $\gamma\delta$ T cell-deficient mice when compared with the wild-type mice [91].

Genomic localisation and creation of TCR diversity

The TCR β and γ chains are encoded by genes located on chromosome 7q35, while the α and δ chains genes are located on chromosome 14q11.2. The TCR $\alpha\beta$ heterodimer confers antigen specificity through the use of different variable (VA, VB), diversity (DB), and junctional (JA, JB) gene segments. These gene segments are initially separate in the (germline) genomic DNA. They undergo somatic rearrangement during thymocyte development, to produce a contiguous V-J exon in case of the A-chain gene, and a contiguous VDJ exon for the B-chain gene [92] (Fig. 4). The large number of gene segments for the TCR loci means that combinatorial diversity can generate many transcriptional permutations. The insertion or deletion of junctional nucleotides creates further diversity [93, 94]. RNA processing results in splicing of a C segment to the exon, which is subsequently translated into glycoprotein chains. Structural consideration suggests that the resulting V-(D)-J junction, which corresponds to the CDR3 region of immunoglobulins, directly contacts antigenic peptides in the MHC peptide-binding site [95]. The T cell recognition of an antigen, and hence its activation, occurs within this specialised area of contact known as the "immunologic synapse", which is localised to areas of glycolipid-enriched membrane micro-domains. T cell activation is dependent not only on specific recognition of the peptide-MHC complex but also on a variety of co-stimulatory receptors and interactions, e.g., CD28 and TNF/TNFR superfamilies [96].

TCR gene polymorphism

Individual TCR gene segments are polymorphic, and many "TCR haplotypes" exist [97]. Most of the polymorphisms are due to allelic variation within the V region gene segments [98,99]. While most of these loci are bi-allelic, some gene segments exhibit more extensive allelism [99]. At least 20% of the genes in the TCR B-gene complex have two alleles or more [100, 101]. Allelic loci have also been found within the TCR AV locus [102–104], which include microsatellites and multiple single nucleotide polymorphisms (SNPs) [105]. Allelic variation that causes amino-acid substitution may alter the receptor's ability to recognise the antigen.

The T cell repertoire

The T cell repertoire is defined as the total population of mature and developing T cells with particular antigen specificities. This repertoire varies between individuals because of the use of different TCR V and J segments [106, 107]. In normal subjects, the peripheral blood TCR repertoire is highly diverse and stable over time. The study of the TCR repertoire in a particular disease may lead to the definition of subsets of T cells expressing a certain V region that could be responsible for the disease, or it may give insight into the nature of the stimulus and mechanisms driving the accumulation of activated T cells. Usage of particular TCR V gene families may induce the development of Th2 sub-type of T cells, which promote IgE production [108]. The pattern of VA or VB gene expression gives an indication of whether non-specific recruitment of T cells is occurring, in which case polyclonal gene expression is seen. Antigen-driven stimulation usually leads to oligoclonal expansion, while the polyclonal expansion of one VB with different antigen specificity may indicate a

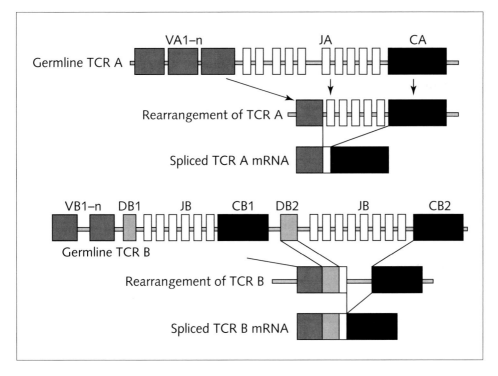

Figure 4
Rearrangement of TCR genes at the germline level and the creation of TCR A and B transcripts.

response to a super-antigen. The identification of a certain V gene expression in disease may lead to the characterisation of antigenic epitopes, with the possibility of using these epitopes as peptides for immunotherapeutic purposes.

Study of the TCR repertoire using monoclonal antibodies against particular V or J segments and flow-cytometry is considered the method of choice, as it is more reproducible than PCR-based methods. However, the number of available clonotypic V antibodies is limited. Few Vα-specific antibodies are available, and about 50% of the Vβ repertoire is covered. Another disadvantage of using monoclonal antibodies is the lack of sequence information, which is required for the study of T-cell clonality. PCR-based techniques could permit a V-region, family-specific PCR (using V-region-specific primers). This method is rapid, but the variation in the efficiency of the PCR, depending on the primer set used, may lead to artefactual results. The anchored PCR method uses one set of primers designed to amplify all the V-J mRNA species and hence overcomes the variability in PCR observed with the family-specific method. In addition, sequencing of the amplified PCR products allows the study of the CDR3 region and hence T cell clonality. In general, however, PCR-based techniques are less reproducible than antibody analysis. Studies will become more reliable as more antibodies against a wider range of Vα and Vβ segments become available and with the advent of more quantitative, reproducible PCR-based methods [109, 110].

Several studies have shown that the repertoire is more stable in the CD4⁺ than in the CD8⁺ subsets of the T cell [111, 112]. The repertoire is influenced by genetic factors, particularly the MHC [113, 114], but during life the repertoire may be modified by a proliferation of T cells responding to antigenic stimulation. TCR AV-segments usage may be under stronger genetic influence than the TCR BV [115]. Twin studies on the TCR AV repertoire showed indistinguishable TCR repertoires between identical twins, but the expressed TCR repertoire can diverge if one of the twins develops an autoimmune disease [115, 116]. In the B6 mouse, polymorphism, in particular TCR AV segments, has a major influence on the MHC restriction of the TCR A repertoire, in which selection of CD4⁺ or CD8⁺ T cell subsets was determined by the complimentarity-determining region 1 (CDR1) or CDR2 preferential interaction with class I and class II MHC molecules [117, 118].

Evidence for a strong *in vivo* selection of particular TCR elements in disease was illustrated in an animal model of experimental allergic encephalitis (EAE), which shares some features of human multiple sclerosis. In this model, murine CD4⁺ T cell clones, which mediate EAE, expressed the same VA4 gene segment, and at least 80% utilised the VB8 gene segment [119]. Immunisation with a synthetic peptide derived from a hypervariable region of the TCR BV8 induced proliferation of Vβ8-specific regulatory T cells, which were found to confer protection against EAE in naive animals [120]. Wedderbun et al. examined the TCR sequences of a panel of HDM-specific T cell clones from an atopic individual with perennial rhinitis using PCR-based techniques [134]. Limited TCR V gene usage was observed, with dominant expression of TCR BV3 and VA8 genes. Similarly, dominant expression of VA13 was observed in the grass allergen *Lol p* I-specific T cell clones [121]. In HLA-DRB1*15 subjects, obtained ragweed allergen *Amb a* V-specific T cell clones showed dominant expression in VB5.2 [122]. The diversity of VA and VB sequences used by T cell clones specific for the major birch tree allergen *Bet v* I was examined in five CD4⁺ T cell clones, each from different individuals, in which all donors possessed the DRB1*07 genotype [123]. Only two of the five clones used an identical VB gene segment, and two clones expressed closely related VA gene segments.

The murine model (BALB/c) of ovalbumin-induced airway hyperreacitivity, which is characterised by the presence of ovalbumin-specific IgE antibodies and cutaneous reactivity to ovalbumin, displayed expansion of TCR BV8S1/8S2 in T cell clones found in the local draining lymph nodes of the airways and lungs [124]. It has been shown that the clinical features of this murine model can be transferred with the transfer of the VB8S1/8S2 positive T cells to naive syngeneic recipients. Mice strain lacking the BV8 subset do not develop the sensitisation to ovalbumin

[124]. Prior sensitisation to the ovalbumin peptide encompassing amino acids 323 through 329 results in the expansion of only BV8S1, indicating that this particular peptide represents the epitope [125]. Treatment of BALB/c mice with antibodies to Vβ8 prior to their sensitisation or bronchial challenge with ovalbumin inhibited the ovalbumin-induced infiltration of eosinophils and airway hyperresponsiveness [126]. Sensitisation of BALB/c mice with ragweed allergen results in a more varied TCR repertoire being expanded (VB8S1,8S2 and VB13) [127]. BALB/c mice also develop aberrant Th2 responses and suffer progressive disease after infection with *Leishmania major*, a response dependent on the production of IL-4 early after infection. One study has demonstrated that the burst of IL-4 mRNA, peaking in draining lymph nodes of BALB/c mice 16 h after infection, occurs within CD4+ T cells that express VB4 VA8 TCRs. VB4-deficient BALB/c mice were resistant to infection. The early IL-4 response was absent in these mice, and Th1 responses occurred following infection. Thus, the IL-4 required for Th2 development and susceptibility to *L. major* is produced by a restricted population of VB4/VA8 CD4+ cells after cognate interaction with a single antigen from this complex organism [128].

The above studies describe the TCR AV/BV gene segments repertoire in synthetic conditions using either *in vitro* T cell clones stimulation or animal models. However, *in vivo* data of TCR V gene segments' repertoire in allergic disease have been limited. Mansur et al. used anchored PCR to quantify the TCR A gene usage at the mRNA level in one atopic individual compared with a normal control [135]. These two individuals shared about 50% of HLA class II genes and both were DRB1*0701 positive. In the atopic individual, the TCR AV gene expression showed excess use of VA1, VA3, and VA8 with evidence for preferential V-J pairing and oligoclonality. In contrast, the normal control displayed random V gene usage. Skewing of TCR AV repertoire secondary to activation of a few T cell clones producing large quantities of mRNA or an expansion within the CD8+ T-cell subset as an explanation for the observed oligoclonality in the atopic subject was not possible to exclude. However, similar results were observed by Gelder et al., who used family PCR to compare the VA gene expression of 8 atopic asthmatics, 8 atopic nonasthmatics, 8 nonatopic nonasthmatics, and 8 nonatopic asthmatics [129]. The TCR AV gene expression was qualitatively estimated by PCR amplification of mRNA extracted from bronchial biopsies and peripheral blood using the VA family-specific primers. Biopsy samples from atopic asthmatic subjects showed mRNA with a mean of 4.8 VA families compared with 11.1 VA families in the nonatopic nonasthmatic group. The pattern of VA family expression in the four groups indicated that the limited expression of the TCR AV families was a characteristic of atopy rather than asthma [129].

Davey et al. analysed the Vβ usage of monozygotic twins discordant for disease using monoclonal antibodies and flow-cytometry technology [112]. Twin pairs discordant for asthma displayed stable differences in Vβ8 and Vβ12 peripheral blood expression. In poorly controlled asthmatics, an increase in Vβ8 in bronchoalveolar lavage fluid (BAL) T cells was seen in both CD4+ and CD8+ subsets, leading to the suggestion that super-antigens are a potential trigger of T cell activation [130]. Yurovsky et al. used family PCR to study VA and VB families in peripheral blood and BAL fluids before and after ragweed challenge in the lungs [131]. Ragweed challenge led to polyclonal influx of T cells in the lungs in addition to oligoclonal activation of both CD4+ and CD8+ T cells. Clonal expansion of T cells was also reported in nonatopic asthmatics [132]. Hodges et al. used monoclonal antibodies to analyse the Vβ repertoire in peripheral blood and BAL derived from the lungs of normal and asthmatic individuals [133]. In both the peripheral blood and BAL derived from the normal and asthmatic individuals, the Vβ repertoire did not differ significantly. Certain Vβ families tended to be expressed at low or high levels in both compartments in the CD3+, CD4+, and CD8+ T cell subsets. There was no significant difference observed in the Vβ repertoire between the asthmatics and controls in either the peripheral blood or the lungs. There were also no consistent changes in Vβ expression in either compartment 24 h after allergen challenge to the lungs of atopic asthmatics.

In general, the above experiments suggest that restricted receptor repertoires do exist for T cells specific for aeroallergens. However, the limited number of T cell clones studied and the limited number of individuals included in such studies make the interpretation of such results difficult. Differences in the methods of studying the TCR repertoire have also introduced another confounding factor. The current findings are nonetheless encouraging, in particular with regard to the identification of TCR V or J segments associated with the allergic disease. For example, the association between VA8 and the development of Th2 cells and allergy to HDM antigens may be causal. Usage of VA8 family might induce Th2 subtype of T cells as observed in BALB/c mice, in which a restricted population of VA8+/VB4+ T cells was responsible for the early IL-4 response required for Th2 CD4+ cell development, and hence the susceptibility to *Leishmania major*, after cognate interaction with a single antigen from this complex organism [128]. The VA8 family showed increased expression in HDM-stimulated CD4+ T cell clones [134] and in the peripheral blood repertoire of an atopic individual [135]. This is supported by the observation of strong association between AV8S1 polymorphism (AV8S1*2) and IgE responses to a major antigenic component of the HDM (*Der p* II) in DRB1*1501-positive subjects [136]. The evidence for VA8 thus far remains circumstantial, but, if established, it may act as precedent for extensive research into this region, leading to the identification of VA or other polymorphisms that predispose to the allergic responses.

Linkage/association of the TCR to allergy and asthma

Several population-based studies have explored the relationship between the TCR and allergic disease. Moffatt et al. were the first to report the presence of linkage of

TCR A/D locus to allergic responsiveness [137]. Using affected sib-pair analysis, they conducted a linkage study between IgE responses to allergens and marker FCA.TA1 in the TCR A/D locus on 14q11.2 and a second marker close to TCR B locus on 7q35. Strong genetic linkage was observed between the TCR A/D locus marker and specific and total IgE, but no linkage was observed with the TCR B locus. The strongest linkage observed was with the purified allergens (*Der p* I, *Der p* II, and *Fel d* I), suggesting that this putative locus may primarily modulate susceptibility to specific allergies [137]. Similar genetic linkage was reported between total IgE and the TCR A/D locus in 53 families taken from a random population sample of urban and rural areas of the Southern Black Forest in Germany. However, in the latter study no linkage was observed with the specific IgE responses [138]. The genome screen by the Collaborative Study on the Genetics of Asthma (CSGA) reported genetic linkage of asthma to markers mapped to 14q11.2-13 close to TCR A/D locus in Caucasian families [36]. FCA.TA1 (marker to TCR A/D) was linked to atopy in 53 multiplex asthma families from Southampton in the UK [139]. The TCR A/D locus also showed linkage to asthma and atopy in 693 Hutterites of a single 15-generation pedigree. The latter genome screen showed no linkage with chromosome 7q [38]. Only one study thus far reported linkage with the TCR B locus but not with the TCR A/D locus. Noguchi et al. reported linkage of a marker to the TCR B locus on 7q35 with both total IgE and asthma, but they observed no linkage with a TCR A/D marker [140].

Collectively, the above studies provide strong case for a genetic linkage between the TCR A/D locus and asthma and atopy, which also correlates with the evidence obtained from the studies of the T cell repertoire that showed stronger genetic control exerted over the TCR α chain repertoire. Polymorphism within the TCR A locus may predispose to the development of asthma and allergy. Whether such polymorphism affects primarily the specific IgE responsiveness or modifies the predisposition to general atopic status remains unclear. However, despite reports of linkage, direct evidence to implicate the TCR A itself is currently lacking. Two studies reported negative transmission disequilibrium test (TDT) between FCA.TA1 alleles (within the TCR A/D locus) and IgE responses [137, 139]. This presence of positive linkage and negative TDT may imply that the putative gene is distant from the examined marker or that a high recombination rate within TCR A region precludes disequilibrium between the putative gene and marker. The degree of recombination across the TCR A/D locus seems high [141], while the FCA.TA1 microsatellite has been localised to within a 900 kb yeast artificial chromosome [142]. The lack of direct evidence leaves the argument open and suggests that the putative gene may represent any elements of TCR A/D or indeed any other gene in the locality. The product of TCR D gene forms part of the γ/δ receptor on the surface of TCR γ/δ cells. The localisation of these cells to mucosal surfaces, where allergens initiate IgE responses, could suggest a role in IgE regulation. The mast cell chymase-1, which maps to 14q11.2, was also reported to be associated with eczema [143]. However,

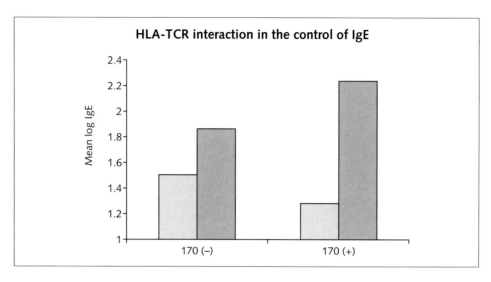

Figure 5

Illustration of the effect of D14S50 allele 170bp interaction on log transformed mean IgE. Hatched area, DRB1*0701 (–) and black area, DRB1*0701 (+) [60].

biologically, the TCR AV genes remain the strongest candidates, particularly when considering their high polymorphic status. This is supported by the observation of association of polymorphism TCR AV8S1*2 and allergy to HDM [136].

HLA/TCR interaction and allergy

Having considered the role HLA and TCR genes individually in asthma and allergy, it is likely that HLA and TCR alleles or molecules interact to modify or restrict the immune response as shown above. Few published population-based studies have addressed the HLA/TCR interaction in relation to the allergic disease. Moffatt et al. examined for an association between the TCR AV8S1 polymorphism (VA8S1*2) and allergy to the purified form of the HDM antigen *Der p* II in context of the HLA-types of all subjects [136]. Sensitisation to *Der p* II was found to be confined to subjects who were positive for VA8S1*2 and HLA-DRB1*1501. These HLA-DR and TCR A alleles, therefore, seem to interact at the germline level to restrict the response to this exogenous antigen [136]. Mansur et al. conducted an association study between HLA/TCR alleles and total serum IgE, with emphasis on whether the HLA/TCR alleles interact to modify total serum IgE [60]. The HLA DRB1*0701 showed strong association with high total IgE, but no allelic association was observed with the D14S50 (marker to TCR A/D). However, a significant interaction was observed between alleles DRB1*0701 and D14S50 such that, when both present, there was a further increase in total serum IgE levels [60] (Fig. 5). In a similar study, D14S50 (allele 170bp) showed association with *Phleum pratense* allergy only in subjects who were DRB1*07 positive [144]. The latter two studies suggest that D14S50 is in linkage disequilibrium with a gene in or close to the TCR A/D locus that interacts with the DRB1*07 allele to increase the IgE responsiveness. The importance of these results is two-fold. First, they show the importance of the combined consideration of the HLA and TCR genes when considering susceptibility loci mapped to these regions. Second, considering the polygenic nature of the genetic predisposition to the allergic disease, the study of HLA/TCR allelic interaction should provide a precedent for more extensive studies of interactions between the different candidate genes for asthma and allergy. Such studies are likely to have more power in dissecting the genetics of the allergic disease, particularly if the modifying environmental factors are accounted for.

Acknowledgement
I would like to acknowledge the contribution of Miss Michelle Plunkett in manuscript preparation and figure design.

References

1   Mosmann TR, Coffman RL (1989) Heterogeneity of cytokine secretion patterns and functions of helper T cells. *Adv Immunol* 46:111–47: 111–147

2   Romagnani S (1992) Human TH1 and TH2 subsets: regulation of differentiation and role in protection and immunopathology. *Int Arch Allergy Immunol* 98: 279–285

3   Sher A, Gazzinelli RT, Oswald IP, Clerici M, Kullberg M, Pearce EJ, Berzofsky JA, Mosmann TR, James SL, Morse HC 3d (1992) Role of T-cell derived cytokines in the down regulation of immune responses in parasitic and retroviral infection. *Immunol Rev* 127: 183–120

4   Plaut M, Pierce JH, Watson CJ, Hanley-Hyde J, Nordan RP, Paul WE (1989) Mast cell lines produce lymphokines in response to cross-linkage of Fc epsilon RI or to calcium ionophores. *Nature* 339: 64–67

5   Bradding P, Feather IH, Howarth PH, Mueller R, Roberts JA, Britten K, Bews JP, Hunt TC, Okayama Y, Heusser CH (1992) Interleukin 4 is localized to and released by human mast cells. *J Exp Med* 176: 1381–1386

6   Prieschl EE, Gouilleux-Gruart V, Walker C, Harrer NE, Baumruker T (1995) A nuclear factor of activated T cell-like transcription factor in mast cells is involved in IL-5 gene regulation after IgE plus antigen stimulation. *J Immunol* 154: 6112–6119

7   Broide DH, Paine MM, Firestein GS (1992) Eosinophils express interleukin 5 and gran-

ulocyte macrophage-colony- stimulating factor mRNA at sites of allergic inflammation in asthmatics. *J Clin Invest* 90: 1414–1424

8   Sousa AR, Poston RN, Lane SJ, Nakhosteen JA, Lee TH (1993) Detection of GM-CSF in asthmatic bronchial epithelium and decrease by inhaled corticosteroids. *Am Rev Respir Dis* 147: 1557–1561

9   Kopf M, Le Gros G, Bachmann M, Lamers MC, Bluethmann H, Kohler G (1993) Disruption of the murine IL-4 gene blocks Th2 cytokine responses. *Nature* 362: 245–248

10   Schwartz RH (1996) Models of T cell anergy: is there a common molecular mechanism? *J Exp Med* 184: 1–8

11   Krummel MF, Allison JP (1995) CD28 and CTLA-4 have opposing effects on the response of T cells to stimulation. *J Exp Med* 182: 459–465

12   Lenschow DJ, Walunas TL, Bluestone JA (1996) CD28/B7 system of T cell costimulation. *Annu Rev Immunol* 14: 233–58

13   McArthur JG, Raulet DH (1993) CD28-induced costimulation of T helper type 2 cells mediated by induction of responsiveness to interleukin 4. *J Exp Med* 178: 1645–1653

14   Vercelli D, Jabara HH, Geha RS (1989) Regulation of human IgE synthesis. *Intern Rev Immunol* 5: 111–115

15   Vercelli D, Jabara HH, Arai K, Geha RS (1989) Induction of human IgE synthesis requires interleukin 4 and T/B cell interactions involving the T cell receptor/CD3 complex and MHC class II antigens. *J Exp Med* 169: 1295–1307

16   Gauchat JF, Gascan H, Roncarolo MG, Rousset F, Pene J, de Vries JE (1991) Regulation of human IgE synthesis: the role of CD4[+] and CD8[+] T-cells and the inhibitory effects of interferon-alpha. *Eur Respir J* (Suppl) 13: 31s–38s

17   Gauchat JF, Mazzei G, Life P, Henchoz S, Peitsch MC, Aubry JP, Jomotte T, Bonnefoy JY (1994) Human CD40 ligand: molecular cloning, cellular distribution and regulation of IgE synthesis. *Research Immunol* 145: 240–244

18   Gauchat JF, Henchoz S, Mazzei G, Aubry JP, Brunner T, Blasey H, Life P, Talabot D, Flores-Romo L, Thompson J et al (1993) Induction of human IgE synthesis in B cells by mast cells and basophils. *Nature* 365: 340–343

19   Schreuder GM, Hurley CK, Marsh SG, Lau M, Maiers M, Kollman C, Noreen H (1999) The HLA dictionary 1999: a summary of HLA-A, -B, -C, -DRB1/3/4/5, -DQB1 alleles and their association with serologically defined HLA-A, -B, -C, -DR, and -DQ antigens. *Hum Immunol* 60: 1157–1181

20   Daar AS, Fuggle SV, Fabre JW, Ting A, Morris PJ (1984) The detailed distribution of HLA-A, B, C antigens in normal human organs. *Transplantation* 38: 287–292

21   Germain RN, Sant AJ, Braunstein NS, Ronchese F (1988) The molecular basis of antigen presentation. *Princess Takamatsu Symp* 19: 179–191

22   Lee JS, Trowsdale J, Travers PJ, Carey J, Grosveld F, Jenkins J, Bodmer WF (1982) Sequence of an HLA-DR alpha-chain cDNA clone and intron-exon organization of the corresponding gene. *Nature* 299: 750–752

23   Brown JH, Jardetzky TS, Gorga JC, Stern LJ, Urban RG, Strominger JL, Wiley DC

(1993) Three-dimensional structure of the human class II histocompatibility antigen HLA-DR1. *Nature* 364: 33–39

24 Daar AS, Fuggle SV, Fabre JW, Ting A, Morris PJ (1984) The detailed distribution of MHC Class II antigens in normal human organs. *Transplantation* 38: 293–298

25 Das HK, Lawrance SK, Weissman SM (1983) Structure and nucleotide sequence of the heavy chain gene of HLA-DR. *Proc Natl Acad Sci USA* 80: 3543–3547

26 Bodmer JG, Marsh SG, Albert ED, Bodmer WF, Dupont B, Erlich HA, Mach B, Mayr WR, Parham P, Sasazuki T (1994) Nomenclature for factors of the HLA system, 1994. *Hum Immunol* 41: 1–20

27 Pascarella S, Argos P (1992) Analysis of insertions/deletions in protein structures. *J Mol Biol* 224: 461–471

28 Bell JI, Todd JA (1989) HLA class II sequences infer mechanisms for major histocompatibility complex-associated disease susceptibility. *Mol Biol Med* 6: 43–53

29 Servenius B, Gustafsson K, Widmark E, Emmoth E, Andersson G, Larhammar D, Rask L, Peterson PA (1984) Molecular map of the human HLA-SB (HLA-DP) region and sequence of an SB alpha (DP alpha) pseudogene. *EMBO J* 3: 3209–3214

30 Le Bouteiller P (1994) HLA class I chromosomal region, genes, and products: facts and questions. *Crit Rev Immunol* 14: 89–129

31 Schmidt CM, Orr HT (1993) Maternal/fetal interactions: the role of the MHC class I molecule HLA-G. *Crit Rev Immunol* 13: 207–224

32 Trowsdale J, Ragoussis J, Campbell RD (1991) Map of the human MHC. *Immunol Today* 12: 443–446

33 Baur MP, Danilovs JA (1980) Reference tables for two and three locus haplotype frequencies of HLA-A, -B, -C, DR, Bf and GLO. In: P Terasaki (ed): *Histocompatibility testing*. Terasaki Press, Los Angeles, 994–1210

34 Hardy DA, Bell JI, Long EO, Lindsten T, McDevitt HO (1986) Mapping of the class II region of the human major histocompatibility complex by pulsed-field gel electrophoresis. *Nature* 323: 453–455

35 Daniels SE, Bhattacharrya S, James A, Leaves NI, Young A, Hill MR, Faux JA, Ryan GF, le Souef PN, Lathrop GM et al (1996) A genome-wide search for quantitative trait loci underlying asthma. *Nature* 383: 247–250

36 The Collaborative Study on the Genetics of Asthma (1997) A genome-wide search for asthma susceptibility loci in ethnically diverse populations. The Collaborative Study on the Genetics of Asthma (CSGA). *Nature Genet* 15: 389–392

37 Hizawa N, Collins G, Rafnar T, Huang SK, Duffy DL, Weber JL, Freidhoff LR, Ehrlich E, Marsh DG, Beaty TH et al (1998) Linkage analysis of Dermatophagoides pteronyssinus-specific IgE responsiveness with polymorphic markers on chromosome 6p21 (HLA-D region) in Caucasian families by the transmission/disequilibrium test. Collaborative Study on the Genetics of Asthma (CSGA). *J Allergy Clin Immunol* 102: 443–448

38 Ober C, Tsalenko A, Parry R, Cox NJ (2000) A second-generation genomewide screen for asthma-susceptibility alleles in a founder population. *Am J Hum Genet* 67: 1154–1162

39 Young RP, Dekker JW, Wordsworth BP, Schou C, Pile KD, Matthiesen F, Rosenberg WM, Bell JI, Hopkin JM, Cookson WO (1994) HLA-DR and HLA-DP genotypes and immunoglobulin E responses to common major allergens. *Clin Exp Allergy* 24: 431–439

40 Stephan V, Kuehr J, Seibt A, Saueressig H, Zingsem S, Dinh TD, Moseler M, Wahn V, Deichmann KA (1999) Genetic linkage of HLA-class II locus to mite-specific IgE immune responsiveness. *Clin Exp Allergy* 29: 1049–1054

41 Kurz T, Strauch K, Heinzmann A, Braun S, Jung M, Ruschendorf F, Moffatt MF, Cookson WO, Inacio F, Ruffilli A et al (2000) A European study on the genetics of mite sensitization. *J Allergy Clin Immunol* 106: 925–932

42 Levine BB, Stember RH, Fotino M (1972) Ragweed hay fever: genetic control and linkage to HL-A haplotypes. *Science* 178: 1201–1203

43 Marsh DG, Meyers DA, Bias WB (1981) The epidemiology and genetics of atopic allergy. *N Engl J Med* 305: 1551–1559

44 Marsh DG, Zwollo P, Huang SK (1991) Molecular and cellular studies of human immune responsiveness to the short ragweed allergen, *Amb a* V. *Eur Respir J* (Suppl) 13: 60s–67s

45 Blumenthal M, Marcus-Bagley D, Awdeh Z, Johnson B, Yunis EJ, Alper CA (1992) HLA-DR2, [HLA-B7, SC31, DR2], and [HLA-B8, SC01, DR3] haplotypes distinguish subjects with asthma from those with rhinitis only in ragweed pollen allergy. *J Immunol* 148: 411–416

46 Tautz C, Rihs HP, Thiele A, Zwollo P, Freidhoff LR, Marsh DG, Baur X (1994) Association of class II sequences encoding DR1 and DQ5 specificities with hypersensitivity to chironomid allergen Chi t I. *J Allergy Clin Immunol* 93: 918–925

47 Donfack J, Tsalenko A, Hoki DM, Parry R, Solway J, Lester LA, Ober C (2000) HLA-DRB1*01 alleles are associated with sensitization to cockroach allergens. *J Allergy Clin Immunol* 105: 960–966

48 Fischer GF, Pickl WF, Fae I, Ebner C, Ferreira F, Breiteneder H, Vikoukal E, Scheiner O, Kraft D (1992) Association between IgE response against *Bet v* I, the major allergen of birch pollen, and HLA-DRB alleles. *Hum Immunol* 33: 259–265

49 Sparholt SH, Georgsen J, Madsen HO, Svendsen UG, Schou C (1994) Association between HLA-DRB3*0101 and immunoglobulin-E responsiveness to *Bet v* I. *Hum Immunol* 39: 76–78

50 Freidhoff LR, Ehrlich-Kautzky E, Meyers DA, Ansari AA, Bias WB, Marsh DG (1988) Association of HLA-DR3 with human immune response to *Lol p* I and *Lol p* II allergens in allergic subjects. *Tissue Antigens* 31: 211–219

51 Ansari AA, Freidhoff LR, Meyers DA, Bias WB, Marsh DG (1989) Human immune responsiveness to Lolium perenne pollen allergen *Lol p* III (rye III) is associated with HLA-DR3 and DR5. *Hum Immunol* 25: 59–71

52 Young RP, Barker RD, Pile KD, Cookson WO, Taylor AJ (1995) The association of HLA-DR3 with specific IgE to inhaled acid anhydrides. *Am J Respir Crit Care Med* 151: 219–221

53 Marsh DG, Blumenthal MN, Ishikawa T, Ruffilli A, Sparholt S, Freidhoff LR (1992)

HLA and specific immune responsiveness to allergens. *Proceedings of Eleventh International Histocompatibility Workshop and Conference*. Oxford University Press, Oxford, Vol. I: 765–776

54   Senechal H, Geny S, Desvaux FX, Busson M, Mayer C, Aron Y, Oster JP, Bessot JC, Peltre G, Pauli G et al (1999) Genetics and specific immune response in allergy to birch pollen and food: evidence of a strong, positive association between atopy and the HLA class II allele HLA-DR7. *J Allergy Clin Immunol* 104: 395–401

55   Chauhan B, Santiago L, Hutcheson PS, Schwartz HJ, Spitznagel E, Castro M, Slavin RG, Bellone CJ (2000) Evidence for the involvement of two different MHC class II regions in susceptibility or protection in allergic bronchopulmonary aspergillosis. *J Allergy Clin Immunol* 106: 723–729

56   Marsh DG, Freidhoff LR, Ehrlich-Kautzky E, Bias WB, Roebber M (1987) Immune responsiveness to *Ambrosia artemisiifolia* (short ragweed) pollen allergen *Amb a* VI (Ra6) is associated with HLA-DR5 in allergic humans. *Immunogenetics* 26: 230–236

57   Cardaba B, Vilches C, Martin E, De Andres B, Del Pozo V, Hernandez D, Gallardo S, Fernandez JC, Villalba M, Rodriguez R (1993) DR7 and DQ2 are positively associated with immunoglobulin-E response to the main antigen of olive pollen (*Ole e* I) in allergic patients. *Hum Immunol* 38: 293–299

58   Cardaba B, De Pablo R, Vilches C, Martin E, Geller-Bernstein C, De Andres B, Zaharan Y, Del Pozo V, Gallardo S, De Arruda Chaves E et al (1996) Allergy to olive pollen: T-cell response from olive allergic patients is restricted by DR7-DQ2 antigens. *Clin Exp Allergy* 26: 316–322

59   Aron Y, Desmazes-Dufeu N, Matran R, Polla BS, Dusser D, Lockhart A, Swierczewski E (1996) Evidence of a strong, positive association between atopy and the HLA class II alleles DR4 and DR7. *Clin Exp Allergy* 26: 821–828

60   Mansur AH, Williams GA, Bishop DT, Markham AF, Lewis S, Britton J, Morrison JF (2000) Evidence for a role of HLA DRB1 alleles in the control of IgE levels, strengthened by interacting TCR A/D marker alleles. *Clin Exp Allergy* 30: 1371–1378

61   Molnar-Gabor E, Endreffy E, Rozsasi A (2000) HLA-DRB1, -DQA1, and -DQB1 genotypes in patients with nasal polyposis. *Laryngoscope* 110: 422–425

62   Cho SH, Kim YK, Oh HB, Jung JW, Son JW, Lee MH, Jee HS, Kim YY, Min KU (2000) Association of HLA-DRB1*07 and DRB1*04 to citrus red mite (*Panonychus citri*) and house dust mite sensitive asthma. *Clin Exp Allergy* 30: 1568–1575

63   Lara-Marquez ML, Yunis JJ, Layrisse Z, Ortega F, Carvallo-Gil E, Montagnani S, Makhatadze NJ, Pocino M, Granja C, Yunis E (1999) Immunogenetics of atopic asthma: association of DRB1*1101 DQA1*0501 DQB1*0301 haplotype with Dermatophagoides spp.-sensitive asthma in a sample of the Venezuelan population. *Clin Exp Allergy* 29: 60–71

64   Howell WM, Standring P, Warner JA, Warner JO (1999) HLA class II genotype, HLA-DR B cell surface expression and allergen specific IgE production in atopic and non-atopic members of asthmatic family pedigrees. *Clin Exp Allergy* 29 (Suppl 4): 35–38

65   Mapp CE, Beghe B, Balboni A, Zamorani G, Padoan M, Jovine L, Baricordi OR, Fab-

bri LM (2000) Association between HLA genes and susceptibility to toluene diiso-cyanate-induced asthma. *Clin Exp Allergy* 30: 651–656

66 Horne C, Quintana PJ, Keown PA, Dimich-Ward H, Chan-Yeung M (2000) Distribu-tion of DRB1 and DQB1 HLA class II alleles in occupational asthma due to western red cedar. *Eur Respir J* 15: 911–914

67 Holloway JW, Doull I, Begishvili B, Beasley R, Holgate ST, Howell WM (1996) Lack of evidence of a significant association between HLA-DR, DQ and DP genotypes and atopy in families with HDM allergy. *Clin Exp Allergy* 26: 1142–1149

68 Dekker JW, Nizankowska E, Schmitz-Schumann M, Pile K, Bochenek G, Dyczek A, Cookson WO, Szczeklik A (1997) Aspirin-induced asthma and HLA-DRB1 and HLA-DPB1 genotypes. *Clin Exp Allergy* 27: 574–577

69 Mullarkey MF, Thomas PS, Hansen JA, Webb DR, Nisperos B (1986) Association of aspirin-sensitive asthma with HLA-DQw2. *Am Rev Respir Dis* 133: 261–263

70 Corrigan CJ (1992) Genetics and regulation of the human immune response. Report on a symposium held at Ringberg Castle, Rottach-Egern a. Tegernsee. *Clin Exp Allergy* 22: 869–875

71 Valenta R, Steinberger P, Duchene M, Kraft D (1996) Immunological and structural sim-ilarities among allergens: prerequisite for a specific and component-based therapy of allergy. *Immunol Cell Biol* 74: 187–194

72 Bignon JS, Aron Y, Ju LY, Kopferschmitt MC, Garnier R, Mapp C, Fabbri LM, Pauli G, Lockhart A, Charron D et al (1994) HLA class II alleles in isocyanate-induced asthma. *Am J Respir Crit Care Med* 149: 71–75

73 Fabbri LM, Mapp CE, Balboni A, Baricordi R (1995) HLA class II molecules and asth-ma induced by toluene diisocyanate. *Int Arch Allergy Immunol* 107: 400–401

74 Turner MW, Brostoff J, Wells RS, Soothill JF (1977) Histocompatibility antigens in atopy with special reference to eczema and hay fever. *Monogr Allergy* 11:19–23

75 Marsh DG, Meyers DA, Freidhoff LR, Hussain R, Hsu SH, Bias WB (1981) Association of HLA phenotypes A1, B8, DW3 and A3, B7, DW2 with allergy. *Int Arch Allergy Appl Immunol* 66 (Suppl 1): 48–50

76 Ostergaard PA, Eriksen J (1979) Association between HLA-A1,B8 in children with extrinsic asthma and IgA deficiency. *Eur J Pediatr* 131: 263–270

77 Rachelefsky G, Park MS, Siegel S, Terasaki PI, Katz R, Saito S (1976) Strong association between B-lymphocyte group-2 specificity and asthma. *Lancet* 2: 1042–1044

78 Turton CW, Morris L, Buckingham JA, Lawler SD, Turner-Warwick M (1979) Histo-compatibility antigens in asthma: population and family studies. *Thorax* 34: 670–676

79 Brenner MB, Trowbridge IS, Strominger JL (1985) Cross-linking of human T cell recep-tor proteins: association between the T cell idiotype beta subunit and the T3 glycopro-tein heavy subunit. *Cell* 40: 183–190

80 Carson GR, Kuestner RE, Ahmed A, Pettey CL, Concino MF (1991) Six chains of the human T cell antigen receptor.CD3 complex are necessary and sufficient for processing the receptor heterodimer to the cell surface. *J Biol Chem* 266: 7883–7887

81 Hall C, Berkhout B, Alarcon B, Sancho J, Wileman T, Terhorst C (1991) Requirements

for cell surface expression of the human TCR/CD3 complex in non-T cells. *Int Immunol* 3: 359–368

82   Brenner MB, McLean J, Dialynas DP, Strominger JL, Smith JA, Owen FL, Seidman JG, Ip S, Rosen F, Krangel MS (1986) Identification of a putative second T-cell receptor. *Nature* 322: 145–149

83   Elliott JF, Rock EP, Patten PA, Davis MM, Chien YH (1988) The adult T-cell receptor delta-chain is diverse and distinct from that of fetal thymocytes. *Nature* 331: 627–631

84   Groh V, Fabbi M, Hochstenbach F, Maziarz RT, Strominger JL (1989) Double-negative (CD4⁻CD8⁻) lymphocytes bearing T-cell receptor alpha and beta chains in normal human skin. *Proc Natl Acad Sci USA* 86: 5059–5063

85   Janeway CA Jr (1988) T-cell development. Accessories or coreceptors? *Nature* 335: 208–210

86   Janis EM, Kaufmann SH, Schwartz RH, Pardoll DM (1989) Activation of gamma delta T cells in the primary immune response to *Mycobacterium tuberculosis. Science* 244: 713–716

87   O'Brien RL, Happ MP, Dallas A, Palmer E, Kubo R, Born WK (1989) Stimulation of a major subset of lymphocytes expressing T cell receptor gamma delta by an antigen derived from *Mycobacterium tuberculosis. Cell* 57: 667–674

88   Pfeffer K, Schoel B, Gulle H, Kaufmann SH, Wagner H (1990) Primary responses of human T cells to mycobacteria: a frequent set of gamma/delta T cells are stimulated by protease-resistant ligands. *Eur J Immunol* 20: 1175–1179

89   Tsuji M, Mombaerts P, Lefrancois L, Nussenzweig RS, Zavala F, Tonegawa S (1994) Gamma delta T cells contribute to immunity against the liver stages of malaria in alpha beta T-cell-deficient mice. *Proc Natl Acad Sci USA* 91: 345–349

90   Holt PG, McMenamin C (1991) IgE and mucosal immunity: studies on the role of intraepithelial Ia + dendritic cells and gamma/delta T-lymphocytes in regulation of T-cell activation in the lung. *Clin Exp Allergy* 21 (Suppl 1): 148–52

91   Zuany-Amorim C, Ruffie C, Haile S, Vargaftig BB, Pereira P, Pretolani M (1998) Requirement for gammadelta T cells in allergic airway inflammation. *Science* 280: 1265–1267

92   Wilson RK, Lai E, Concannon P, Barth RK, Hood LE (1988) Structure, organization and polymorphism of murine and human T-cell receptor alpha and beta chain gene families. *Immunol Rev* 101:149–72

93   Davis MM, Bjorkman PJ (1988) T-cell antigen receptor genes and T-cell recognition. *Nature* 334: 395–402

94   Hedrick SM, Engel I, McElligott DL, Fink PJ, Hsu ML, Hansburg D, Matis LA (1988) Selection of amino acid sequences in the beta chain of the T cell antigen receptor. *Science* 239: 1541–1544

95   Jorgensen JL, Esser U, Fazekas de St.Groth B, Reay PA, Davis MM (1992) Mapping T-cell receptor-peptide contacts by variant peptide immunization of single-chain transgenics. *Nature* 355: 224–230

96 Salazar-Fontana LI, Bierer BE (2000) T-lymphocyte coactivator molecules. *Curr Opin Hematol* 8: 5–11

97 Concannon P, Gatti RA, Hood LE (1987) Human T cell receptor V beta gene polymorphism. *J Exp Med* 165: 1130–1140

98 Cornelis F, Pile K, Loveridge J, Moss P, Harding R, Julier C, Bell J (1993) Systematic study of human alpha beta T cell receptor V segments shows allelic variations resulting in a large number of distinct T cell receptor haplotypes. *Eur J Immunol* 23: 1277–1283

99 Gomolka M, Epplen C, Buitkamp J, Epplen JT (1993) Novel members and germline polymorphisms in the human T-cell receptor Vb6 family. *Immunogenetics* 37: 257–265

100 Barron KS, Deulofeut H, Robinson MA (1995) TCRBV20S1 allele frequencies vary among human populations. *Immunogenetics* 41: 383–385

101 Deulofeut H, Wilderson JL, Barron KS, Robinson MA (1995) TCRBV12 genes are polymorphic but the protein products encoded by each gene are conserved. *Hum Immunol* 43: 227–230

102 Wright AL, Holberg C, Martinez FD, Taussig LM (1991) Relationship of parental smoking to wheezing and nonwheezing lower respiratory tract illnesses in infancy. Group Health Medical Associates. *J Pediatr* 118: 207–214

103 Reyburn H, Cornelis F, Russell V, Harding R, Moss P, Bell J (1993) Allelic polymorphism of human T-cell receptor V alpha gene segments. *Immunogenetics* 38: 287–291

104 Moody AM, Reyburn H, Willcox N, Newsom-Davis J (1998) New polymorphism of the human T-cell receptor AV28S1 gene segment. *Immunogenetics* 48: 62–64

105 Moffatt MF, Traherne JA, Abecasis GR, Cookson WO (2000) Single nucleotide polymorphism and linkage disequilibrium within the TCR alpha/delta locus. *Hum Mol Genet* 9: 1011–1019

106 Chothia C, Boswell DR, Lesk AM (1988) The outline structure of the T-cell alpha beta receptor. *EMBO J* 7: 3745–3755

107 Rosenberg WM, Moss PA, Bell JI (1992) Variation in human T cell receptor V beta and J beta repertoire: analysis using anchor polymerase chain reaction. *Eur J Immunol* 22: 541–549

108 Heinzel FP, Sadick MD, Mutha SS, Locksley RM (1991) Production of interferon gamma, interleukin 2, interleukin 4, and interleukin 10 by CD4+ lymphocytes *in vivo* during healing and progressive murine leishmaniasis. *Proc Natl Acad Sci USA* 88: 7011–7015

109 Muraro PA, Jacobsen M, Necker A, Nagle JW, Gaber R, Sommer N, Oertel WH, Martin R, Hemmer B (2000) Rapid identification of local T cell expansion in inflammatory organ diseases by flow cytometric T cell receptor V beta analysis. *J Immunol Methods* 246: 131–143

110 Yoshida R, Yoshioka T, Yamane S, Matsutani T, Toyosaki-Maeda T, Tsuruta Y, Suzuki R (2000) A new method for quantitative analysis of the mouse T-cell receptor V region repertoires: comparison of repertoires among strains. *Immunogenetics* 52: 35–45

111 Hawes GE, Struyk L, van den Elsen PJ (1993) Differential usage of T cell receptor V

gene segments in CD4+ and CD8+ subsets of T lymphocytes in monozygotic twins. *J Immunol* 150: 2033–2045

112 Davey MP, Meyer MM, Bakke AC (1994) T cell receptor V beta gene expression in monozygotic twins. Discordance in CD8 subset and in disease states. *J Immunol* 152: 315–321

113 Akolkar PN, Gulwani-Akolkar B, Pergolizzi R, Bigler RD, Silver J (1993) Influence of HLA genes on T cell receptor V segment frequencies and expression levels in peripheral blood lymphocytes. *J Immunol* 150: 2761–2773

114 Gulwani-Akolkar B, Akolkar PN, McKinley M, Fisher SE, Silver J (1995) Crohn's disease is accompanied by changes in the CD4+, but not CD8+, T cell receptor BV repertoire of lamina propria lymphocytes. *Clin Immunol Immunopathol* 77: 95–106

115 Moss PA, Rosenberg WM, Zintzaras E, Bell JI (1993) Characterization of the human T cell receptor alpha-chain repertoire and demonstration of a genetic influence on V alpha usage. *Eur J Immunol* 23: 1153–1159

116 Moss PA, Rosenberg WM, Bell JI (1992) The human T cell receptor in health and disease. *Annu Rev Immunol* 10: 71–96

117 Sim BC, Zerva L, Greene MI, Gascoigne NRJ (1996) Control of MHC restriction by TCR Valpha CDR1 and CDR2. *Science* 273: 963–966

118 Torres-Nagel N, Mehling B, LeRolle AF, Joly E, Hunig T (2000) Genetic control of peripheral TCRAV usage by representation in the preselection repertoire and MHC allele-specific overselection. *Int Immunol* 13: 63–73

119 Acha-Orbea H, Mitchell DJ, Timmermann L, Wraith DC, Tausch GS, Waldor MK, Zamvil SS, McDevitt HO, Steinman L (1988) Limited heterogeneity of T cell receptors from lymphocytes mediating autoimmune encephalomyelitis allows specific immune intervention. *Cell* 54: 263–273

120 Vandenbark AA, Hashim G, Offner H (1989) Immunization with a synthetic T-cell receptor V-region peptide protects against experimental autoimmune encephalomyelitis. *Nature* 341: 541–544

121 Mohapatra SS (1994) Determinant spreading: implications in allergic disorders. *Immunol Today* 15: 596–597

122 Huang SK, Xiao HQ, Kleine-Tebbe J, Paciotti G, Marsh DG, Lichtenstein LM, Liu MC (1995) IL-13 expression at the sites of allergen challenge in patients with asthma. *J Immunol* 155: 2688–2694

123 Breiteneder H, Scheiner O, Hajek R, Hulla W, Huttinger R, Fischer G, Kraft D, Ebner C (1995) Diversity of TCRAV and TCRBV sequences used by human T-cell clones specific for a minimal epitope of Bet v 1, the major birch pollen allergen. *Immunogenetics* 42: 53–58

124 Renz H, Gelfand EW (1992) T-cell receptor V elements regulate murine IgE production and airways responsiveness. *Allergy* 47: 270–276

125 Renz H, Bradley K, Saloga J, Loader J, Larsen GL, Gelfand EW (1993) T cells expressing specific V beta elements regulate immunoglobulin E production and airways responsiveness *in vivo*. *J Exp Med* 177: 1175–1180

126 Hofstra CL, Van Ark I, Savelkoul HF, Cruikshank WW, Nijkamp FP, Van Oosterhout AJ (1998) Vbeta8+ T lymphocytes are essential in the regulation of airway hyperresponsiveness and bronchoalveolar eosinophilia but not in allergen-specific IgE in a murine model of allergic asthma. *Clin Exp Allergy* 28: 1571–1580

127 Renz H, Bradley K, Larsen GL, McCall C, Gelfand EW (1993) Comparison of the allergenicity of ovalbumin and ovalbumin peptide 323– 339. Differential expansion of V beta-expressing T cell populations. *J Immunol* 151: 7206–7213

128 Launois P, Maillard I, Pingel S, Swihart KG, Xenarios I, Acha-Orbea H, Diggelmann H, Locksley RM, MacDonald HR, Louis JA (1997) IL-4 rapidly produced by V beta 4 V alpha 8 CD4+ T cells instructs Th2 development and susceptibility to Leishmania major in BALB/c mice. *Immunity* 6: 541–549

129 Gelder CM, Morrison JF, Chung KF, Barnes PJ, Adcock IM (1996) T cell receptor repertoire in peripheral blood and bronchial biopsies from normal and asthmatic subjects. *Biochem Soc Trans* 24: 316S

130 Hauk PJ, Wenzel SE, Trumble AE, Szefler SJ, Leung DY (1999) Increased T-cell receptor vbeta8+ T cells in bronchoalveolar lavage fluid of subjects with poorly controlled asthma: a potential role for microbial superantigens. *J Allergy Clin Immunol* 104: 37–45

131 Yurovsky VV, Weersink EJ, Meltzer SS, Moore WC, Postma DS, Bleecker ER, White B (1998) T-Cell repertoire in the blood and lungs of atopic asthmatics before and after ragweed challenge. *Am J Respir Cell Mol Biol* 18: 370–383

132 Umibe T, Kita Y, Nakao A, Nakajima H, Fukuda T, Yoshida S, Sakamaki T, Saito Y, Iwamoto I (2000) Clonal expansion of T cells infiltrating in the airways of non-atopic asthmatics. *Clin Exp Immunol* 119: 390–397

133 Hodges E, Dasmahapatra J, Smith JL, Quin CT, Lanham S, Krishna MT, Holgate ST, Frew AJ (1998) T cell receptor (TCR) Vbeta gene usage in bronchoalveolar lavage and peripheral blood T cells from asthmatic and normal subjects. *Clin Exp Immunol* 112: 363–374

134 Wedderburn LR, O'Hehir RE, Hewitt CR, Lamb JR, Owen MJ (1993) *In vivo* clonal dominance and limited T-cell receptor usage in human CD4+ T-cell recognition of house dust mite allergens. *Proc Natl Acad Sci USA* 90: 8214–8218

135 Mansur AH, Gelder CM, Holland D, Campbell DA, Griffin A, Cunliffe W, Markham AF, Morrison JF (1996) Non random usage of T cell receptor alpha gene expression in atopy using anchored PCR. *Adv Exp Med Biol* 409:381–389

136 Moffatt MF, Schou C, Faux JA, Cookson WO (1997) Germline TCR-A restriction of immunoglobulin E responses to allergen. *Immunogenetics* 46: 226–230

137 Moffatt MF, Hill MR, Cornelis F, Schou C, Faux JA, Young RP, James AL, Ryan G, le Souef P, Musk AW et al (1994) Genetic linkage of T-cell receptor alpha/delta complex to specific IgE responses. *Lancet* 343: 1597–1600

138 Deichmann KA, Hildebrandt F, Kuehr J, Forster J (1995) Genetic linkage analysis of predicted asthma genes and atopy. *Allergy* 50 (Suppl): 164

139 Mansur AH, Bishop DT, Markham AF, Morton NE, Holgate ST, Morrison JF (1999)

Suggestive evidence for genetic linkage between IgE phenotypes and chromosome 14q markers. *Am J Respir Crit Care Med* 159: 1796–1802

140 Noguchi E, Shibasaki M, Arinami T, Takeda K, Yokouchi Y, Kawashima T, Yanagi H, Matsui A, Hamaguchi H (1998) Association of asthma and the interleukin-4 promoter gene in Japanese. *Clin Exp Allergy* 28: 449–453

141 Robinson MA, Kindt TJ (1987) Genetic recombination within the human T-cell receptor alpha-chain gene complex. *Proc Natl Acad Sci USA* 84: 9089–9093

142 Cornelis F, Hashimoto L, Loveridge J, MacCarthy A, Buckle V, Julier C, Bell J (1992) Identification of a CA repeat at the TCRA locus using yeast artificial chromosomes: a general method for generating highly polymorphic markers at chosen loci. *Genomics* 13: 820–825

143 Mao XQ, Shirakawa T, Yoshikawa T, Yoshikawa K, Kawai M, Sasaki S, Enomoto T, Hashimoto T, Furuyama J, Hopkin JM et al (1996) Association between genetic variants of mast-cell chymase and eczema. *Lancet* 348: 581–583

144 Moffatt MF, Young A, Schou C, Faux JA, Musk AW, Cookson WO (1995) Involvement of TCR alpha/delta and HLA-DR in specific allergy. *Allergy* 50 (Suppl): 164

Chromosome 11q13, FcεRIβ and atopic asthma

Chaker N. Adra[1], X.-Q. Mao[2,3], A. Yamasaki[2], P.-S. Gao[3], Xing Yang[1,3], T. Shirakawa[2,3] and J.M. Hopkin[3]

[1]Beth Israel Deaconess Medical Center, Harvard Medical School, Boston, MA 02215, USA; [2]Department of Health Promotion and Human Behavior, Kyoto University Graduate School of Public Health, Kyoto 606-8501, Japan; [3]Experimental Medicine Unit, University of Swansea, Swansea, UK

Original linkage to chromosome 11q13

Atopy is a common disorder characterized by increased general IgE responsiveness [1]. Atopy is also an important cause of disorder in the skin (eczema), lungs (asthma), and nose (rhinitis); family studies suggest variable combinations of organ-specific clinical syndromes in individuals within atopic families [1–10].

The first genetic region reported to show linkage to atopy was chromosome 11q13 [1, 2]. Data from Japan [3] and Germany [4] using lod scores and from the Netherlands [5] using affected sib-pair methods have confirmed linkage in families with marked atopy irrespective of clinical symptoms. However, a number of studies failed to find linkage to the same region [11–17]. This failure resulted in part because of small sample sizes, differing recruitment strategies and statistical analyses, and the presence of substantial genetic heterogeneity underlying atopy.

The evidence for genetic linkage was further confounded by the existence of a maternal pattern of inheritance [2, 6]. A significant portion of atopic asthmatic families in Caucasian and Japanese populations may be linked to chromosome 11q13 through the maternal line [2, 6]. A maternal pattern of inheritance has been seen in genetic studies of chromosome 11q13 markers in at least five independent studies [2, 6, 10, 18–20]. For some time, it has been recognized that a child has a greater risk of developing atopy if his or her mother is affected as opposed to the father. Similar parent-of-origin effects have been seen in other diseases [21]. These unexpected results imply that both parental phenotypes can influence the effects of the chromosome 11q13 locus. Chromosome 11q13 is not the only locus that has shown maternal effects on the transmission of atopic traits [22], and it will be interesting to see what is revealed when the genetic data for other loci are analyzed further. Certainly, for chromosome 11q13, the results cannot be explained either on the basis of known genetic mechanisms, such as imprinting, or by maternal/fetal interactions.

The Hereditary Basis of Allergic Diseases, edited by Stephen T. Holgate and John W. Holloway
© 2002 Birkhäuser Verlag Basel/Switzerland

Candidate gene *FCER1B* (high affinity IgE receptor β subunit gene)

The β subunit of the high affinity IgE receptor (FcεRIβ) gene has been mapped to chromosome 11q13.1 [8, 9, 23–25] and is a candidate gene for atopy because of its important role in initiating type I allergic reaction by mast cells and basophils. A recent large-scale population-based linkage study, by sib-pair methodology, affirms linkage of asthma with microsatellite repeats of FcεRIβ, but not with outside markers on 11q13 in an Australian population [4].

The FcεRIβ gene is composed of seven exons and six introns, spanning approximately 11 kb [26]. Eight variants of this gene have been identified, including three coding and five non-coding variants; three coding polymorphisms within the *FCER1B* are Ile181Leu, Val183Leu [27–29], and Glu237Gly [30, 31]. A strong association was seen between the 181Leu allele and measures of atopy in a small random sample of 163 subjects. Similarly, in a set of unrelated nuclear families with allergic asthmatic probands, strong association with atopy was found with a maternal pattern of inheritance. The 183Leu allele was not found in either set of subjects. In a larger study of a random population of 1000 subjects, the 181Leu allele was only present in individuals carrying the 183Leu allele. The combination of alleles at amino acids 181 and 183 is referred to as the 181Leu/183Leu allele and was found in only 4% of the subjects. Furthermore, detection of the 181Leu and 181Leu/183Leu alleles has been technically difficult and, in other atopic European populations, neither variant has been found [32, 33]. The low frequency of the 181Leu and the compound 181Leu/183Leu alleles make their significance as atopy-susceptible alleles in European populations questionable, while another Italian group identified Leu181/Leu183 double mutations in a Sardinian population by sequencing [34].

On the other hand, the 181Leu/183Leu allele was found at high frequency (72%) in Kuwaiti Arabs and was associated with asthma, suggesting that it may be an important risk factor in this population [35]. In a study of South African blacks and whites, 181Leu was detected at a high incidence using the amplification refractory mutation system (ARMS), which relies on the specific amplification of each allele [36]. When compared with appropriate control subjects, an association of 181Leu in white South African asthmatics was seen, although no association between black asthmatics and black control subjects was detected. When the 181Leu positive individuals were sequenced, however, only the wild-type sequence (Ile181) was seen. This observation therefore puts into question the validity of this study and reiterates the prior observation that detection of these variants is technically difficult.

A third coding polymorphism in the *FCER1B* gene, called Glu237gGly, has been found at a low frequency (5%) in a number of populations [30, 31]. In Caucasians, significant associations between 237Gly with bronchial hyper-responsiveness (BHR) and skin test responses to grass and house dust-mite allergies have been reported [30]. The 237Gly allele occurs at a high frequency in Japanese asthmatics (20%)

[31] and is associated with atopic asthma, in particular, childhood asthma, as well as with high total serum IgE levels. Personal communications from two independent Japanese groups confirmed genetic association with atopy.

Two additional polymorphisms that do not alter the amino-acid sequence of the protein have also been identified within these genes (Rsal_in2 [37] and Rsal_ex7 [38]). Although these do not have any functional consequences, they have shown strong associations with atopic eczema and asthma in a study of families recruited through a child affected with eczema [39, 40]. Furthermore, a single nucleotide polymorphism in the promoter region is also strongly associated with atopy [41]. A number of studies therefore implicate the *FCER1B* gene as having an influence on the pathogenesis of allergic disease.

A growing body of evidence supports the candidacy of FcεRIβ as an atopy locus; however, the functional action of FcεRIβ variants in promoting atopy remains undefined [42]. A direct functional link of the coding variant, Leu181, in FcεRIβ gene was hypothesized; however, neither significant upregulation of histamine release from basophils [28, 43] nor of phosphorylation of the receptors has been found [44]. More recently, the function of human FcεRIβ has been described more precisely; it amplifies the intensity of cell activation signals through the FcεRIγ chain with a gain of 5- to 7-fold when it couples with FcεRI αγ receptors *in vitro* [45, 46] and *in vivo* [47]. This "amplifier" function is of particular interest because of several non-coding polymorphisms [37–39] that might relate to expression levels of this gene. Further molecular biochemical studies are needed to test whether these polymorphisms are responsible for quantitative change in FcεRIβ's amplifying signals in basophils and mast cells among atopic subjects. More recently, it is demonstrated that FcεRIβ has a second amplification function [48]: the amplification of FcεRI cell surface expression. This funtion is due to an early association of FcεRIβ with Fcε–RIα, resulting in improved traficking and maturation of FcεRIα and receptor complexes. These data provide a possible molecular explanation for the large difference in FcεRI density between FcεRIβ-negative cells such as monocytes, dendritic cells, and FcεRIβ-positive effector cells such as mast cells and basophils. In FcεRIβ positive effector cells, the combined signalling and expression amplification results in an estimated 12- to 30-fold amplification of downstream events.

Another explanation is that an unrecognized atopy gene sits close to FcεRIβ and its variants associate tightly with those of FcεRIβ. A new member of the CD20/FcεRIβ family, the HTm4 gene, has been cloned [49], and recent fine-mapping enables us to determine the distance between FcεRIβ and HTm4 to less than 70 Kb (Adra et al., submitted). HTm4 spans about 13 Kb: the high structural and topological homology (24–60% at transmembranous portions) to CD20 and FcεRIβ enables us to propose that HTm4, FcεRIβ, and CD20 evolved from the same ancestral gene to form a family of four-transmembrane proteins [49] consists of seven exons – a structure quite similar to that of FcεRIβ (Adra et al., submitted). A Taq I restriction fragment length polymorphism (RFLP) in the third intron of the gene was identified, and it showed a strong association with atopic asthma. Since this variant showed similar odds ratio for marked asthma as well as marked atopy phenotypes to those for the intron 2 of the FcεRIβ gene [50], HTm4 might be regarded as a candidate locus for atopy on 11q13.1. Another possibility is that there is an unknown gene between the two genes, FcεRIβ and HTm4, at which variants confer the atopy phenotype. Further physical and functional mapping is under way in our laboratories.

Other loci on 11q13

The second locus for asthma on 11q13.1 is close to D11S480/D11S1883 approximately 5 cM telomeric to FcεRIβ (Fig. 1). We have previously shown strong linkage with clinical symptoms, e.g., asthma at D11S480 in 40 British asthmatic families, but not with atopy phenotype (Dubowitz et al, unpublished data). In this study one of the alleles of D11S480 was associated with marked asthma, but not with any combination of atopy phenotype. These findings suggest that a clinical asthma locus may be localized in close relation to D11S480 independently of FcεRIβ/HTm4 locus on 11q13.1.

The autosomal recessive disorder Bardet-Biedl Syndrome (BBS), which is characterized by retinal degeneration, polydactyly, obesity, mental retardation, hypogenitalism, renal dysplasia, and short stature, is heterogeneous with at least four loci (BBS 1–4) to date [51]. Almost half of our Caucasian families have been linked to 11q13.1 (BBS1) and the highest lods were found at D11S1883 with no recombination. Interestingly, a quarter of our patients linked to BBS1 showed atopic asthma [51]. This indicates that BBS1 might be in linkage disequilibrium with an atopic asthma locus between D11S480 and PYGM (Fig. 1).

More recently, strong genetic association was found between childhood asthma and CC16 [52], 1 cM centromeric to D11S480 on 11q13.1. Biallelic and microsatellite variants have been identified in this gene. The gene for Clara cell secretory protein, CC16, is a plausible candidate because of its involvement in the control of airway inflammation. Protein studies have revealed significant differences in levels between asthmatics and healthy controls. The three exons of CC16 were scanned for polymorphisms in an unselected population of subjects from a set of families and a cohort of severely asthmatic children, both from Perth, Western Australia. A single nt substitution, guanine for adenine, was found at nt 38 in exon 1 (38 A/G). A case-control study of 46 unaffected and 67 asthmatic subjects revealed a significantly higher frequency of the 38A allele in asthmatics compared with unaffected subjects. Homozygotes for the 38A allele had a 6.9-fold increased risk for asthma ($p = 0.049$, 95% CI: 1.01–47.43), whereas heterozygotes (38AG) had a 4.2-fold risk.

These findings have yet to be confirmed, and a subsequent study of the CC16 polymorphism in British [53] and Japanese [54] populations failed to find an association between atopic asthma and the 38A/T genotypes. A previous study by the same group had also failed to find association between asthma and an intragenic microsatellite of *CC16*. Whether variation in the *CC16* gene is a genetic cause of asthma and it accounts for some of the reported linkages on chromosome 11q13 therefore remains to be established. Another candidate is CHRM1 [55], a muscarinic receptor on airways; however, no association was found in our population [50]. Since our patients show no association with D11S1883, data on this study, on BBS1, and on *CC16* suggest that the locus for asthma might be localized close to D11S480.

A third atopic asthma locus on 11q13.1 has been reported telomeric to FGF3, more than 10–12 cM away from FcεRIβ: genetic linkage or association for atopic asthma has been found on 11q13.1 with other markers: *FGF3* [56], D11S534 [57], or D11S97 [58] in relation to total serum IgE level, or D11S527 [57] in relation to asthma or bronchial hyperresponsiveness. Others have found neither association nor linkage for atopic asthmatic phenotypes with any genes or markers on 11q13.1 region [59, 60]. This area of research therefore still remains controversial because of genetic heterogeneity or differences in phenotype assignments among researchers.

References

1   Cookson WOCM, Sharp P, Faux JA, Hopkin JM (1989) Linkage between immunoglobulin E responses underlying asthma and rhinitis, and chromosome 11q. *Lancet* 1: 1292–1295

2   Cookson WOCM, Young RP, Sandford AJ, Moffatt MF, Shirakawa T, Faux JA, Nakamura Y, Cecier J, Rathrop GM, Hopkin JM (1992) Maternal inheritance of atopic IgE responsiveness on chromosome 11q. *Lancet* 340: 381–384

3   Shirakawa T, Hashimoto T, Furuyama J, Morimoto K (1994) Linkage between severe atopy and chromosoem 11q13 in Japanese families. *Clin Genet* 46: 125–130

4   Folster-Holst R, Moises HW, Yang L, Fritsch W, Weissenbach J, Christophers E (1998) Linkage between atopy and the IgE high-affinity receptor gene at 11q13 in atopic dermatitis families. *Hum Genetics* 102: 236–239

5   Collee JM, ten Kate LP, de Vries HG, Kliphuis JW, Scheffer H, Gerritsen J (1993) Allele sharing on chromosome 11q13 in sibs with asthma and atopy. *Lancet* 342: 936

6   Sandford AJ, Shirakawa T, Moffatt MF, Faux JA, Sharp P, Young RP, Ra C, Nakamura Y, Cookson WOCM, Hopkin JM (1993) Localisation of atopy and β subunit of high affinity IgE receptor(FcεRIβ) on chromosome 11q. *Lancet* 341: 332–334

7   Van Herwerden L, Harrap SB, Wong ZYH, Abramson MJ, Forbes AB, Raven J, Lanigan A, Walters EH (1995) Linkage of high-affinity IgE receptor gene with bronchial hyperreactivity, even in absence of atopy. *Lancet* 346: 1262–1265

8   Young RP, Sharp P, Lynch J, Faux JA, Lathrop GM, Cookson WOCM, Hopkin JM (1992) Confirmation of genetic linkage between atopic IgE responses and chromosome 11q13. *J Med Genet* 29: 236–238

9   Moffatt MF, Sharp PA, Faux JA, Young RP, Cookson WOCM, Hopkin JM (1992) Factors confounding genetic linkage between atopy and chromosome 11q. *Clin Exp Allergy* 22: 1046–1051

10 Daniels SE, Bhattacharrya S, James A, Leaves N, Young A, Hill MR, Faux JA, Ryan GF, leSouf PN, Lathrop GM, Musk AW, Cookson WOCM (1996) A genome-wide search for quantitative trait loci underlying asthma. *Nature* 383: 247–250

11 Amelung PJ, Postma DS, Xu J, Meyers DA, Bleecker ER (1998) Exclusion of chromosome 11q and the FcεRI-beta gene as etiologic factor in allergy and asthma in a population of Dutch asthmatic families. *Clin Exp Allergy* 28: 397–403

12 Hizawa N, Yamaguchi E, Ohe M, Itoh A, Furuya K, Ohnuma N, Kawakami Y (1992) Lack of linkage between atopy and chromosome 11q. *Clin Exp Allergy* 22: 1065–1092

13 Limpany P, Welsh KI, Cochrane GM, Kemeny DM, Lee TH (1992) Genetic analysis of the linkage between chromosome 11q and atopy. *Clin Exp Allergy* 22: 1085–1092

14 Rich SS, Roitman-Johnson B, Greenberg B, Roberts S, Blumenthal MN (1992) Genetic analysis of atopy in three large kindreds; no evidence of linkage to D11S97. *Clin Exp Allergy* 22: 1070–1076

15 Noguchi E, Shibasaki M, Arinamai T, Takeda K, Maki T, Miyamoto T, Kawashima T, Kobayashi K, Hamaguchi H (1997) Evidence for linkage between asthma/atopy in childhood and chromosome 5q31-q33 in a Japanese population. *Am J Respir Crit Care Med* 156: 1390–1393

16 Ulbrecht M, Eisenhut T, Bonisch J, Kruse R, Wjst M, Heinrich J, Wichmann H-E, Weiss EH, Albert ED (1997) High serum IgE concentrations: Association with HLA-DR and markers on chromosome 5q31 and chromosome 11q13. *J Allergy Clin Immunol* 99: 828–832

17 Breton HM, Ruffin RE, Thompson PJ, Turner DR (1994) Familial atopy in Australian pedigrees: adventitious linkage to chromosome 8 is not confirmed nor is there evidence of linkage to the high affinity IgE receptor. *Clin Exp Allergy* 24: 868–877

18 Mao X-Q, Shirakawa T, Sasaki S, Enomoto T, Morimoto K, Hopkin J,M (1996) Maternal inheritance of atopy at the FcεRIβ locus in Japanese sibs. *Hum Heredity* 47: 178–180

19 Deichmann KA, Starke B, Schlenther S, Heinzmann A, Sparholt SH, Forster J, Kuehr J (1996) Linkage and association studies of atopy and the chromosome 11q13 region. *J Med Genet* 36: 379–382

20 Martinati LC, Trabetti E, Casartelli A, Boner AL, Pignatti PF (1996) Affected sib-pair and mutation analyses of the high affinity IgE receptor b chain locus in Italian families with atopic asthmatic children. *Am J Respir Crit Care Med* 153: 1682–1685

21 Moffatt MF, Cookson WOCM (1998) The genetics of asthma Maternal effects in atopic disease. *Clin Exp Allergy* 28: 56–66

22 Meyers DA, Marsh DG (1992) Genetics of atopy. In: RA King, JI Rotter, AG Motulsky (eds): *Allergy and asthma*. Oxford University Press, New York, 130

23 Szepetowski P, Gaudray P (1994) *FCERIB*, a candidate gene for atopy, is located in 11q13 between CD20 and TCN1. *Genomics* 19: 399–400

24   Starfford AN, Rider SH, Hopkin JM, Cookson WOCM, Monaco AP (1994) A 28 Mb YAC contig in 11q12-q13 localizes candidate genes for atopy: FcεRIβ, CD20. *Hum Mol Genet* 3: 779–785

25   Sandford AJ, Moffatt MF, Daniels DE, Nakamura Y, Lathrop GM, Hopkin JM, Cookson WOCM (1995) A genetic map of chromosome 11q, including the atopy locus. *Eur J Hum Genet* 3: 188–194

26   Kuster H, Zhang L, Brini AT, MacGlashan DWJ, Kinet J-P (1992) The gene and cDNA for the human high affinity immunoglobulin E receptor beta chain and expression of the complete human receptor. *J Biol Chem* 267: 12782–12787

27   Shirakawa T, Li A, Dubowitz M, Dekker JW, Shaw AE, Faux JA, Ra C, Cookson WOCM, Hopkin JM (1994) Association between atopy and variants of the β subunit of high affinity immunoglobulin E receptor. *Nat Genet* 7: 125–130

28   Li A, Hopkin JM (1997) Atopy phenotype in subjects with variants of the β subunit of the high affinity IgE receptor. *Thorax* 52: 654–655

29   Hill MR, James AL, Faux JA, Ryan G, Hopkin JM, leSouef P, Musk AW, Cookson WOCM (1995) FcεRIβ polymorphism and risk of atopy in a general population. *Br Med J* 311: 776–779

30   Hill MR, Cookson WOCM (1996) A novel coding polymorphism of the C-terminal in FcεRIβ is associated with atopy and bronchial hyper-responsiveness. *Hum Mol Genet* 5: 959–962

31   Shirakawa T, Mao X-Q, Sasaki S, Kawai M, Enomoto T, Hopkin JM, Morimoto K (1996) Associatin between atopic asthma and a coding variant of FcεRIβ in a Japanese population. *Hum Mol Genet* 5: 1129–1130

32   Deichmann KA, Hildebrandt F, Heinzmann A (1996) Absence of mutations in the 6th exon of FcεRIβ. *Adv Exp Med Biol* 409: 355–358

33   Kofler H, Aichberger S, Ott G, Casari A, Kofler R (1996) Lack of association between atopy and the Ile181leu variants of the beta-subunit of the high affinity immunoglobulin E receptor. *Int Arch Allergy Immunol* 111: 44–47

34   Rigoli L, Salpietro DC, Lavelle G, Cafiero G, Zuccarello D, Barberi I (2000) Allelic association of gene markers on chromosome 11q in Italian families with atopy. *Acta Peadiatr* 89: 1056–1061

35   Hijazi Z, Haider MZ, Khan MR, Al-Dowaisan AA (1998) High frequency of IgE receptor FcεRIβ variant(Leu181/Leu183) in Kuwaiti Arabs and its association with asthma. *Clin Genet* 53: 149–152

36   Green SL, Gaillard MC, Song E, Dewar JB, Halkas A (1998) Polymorphisms of the b chain of the high-affinity immunoglobulin E receptor (FcεRIβ) in South African black and white asthmatic and nonasthmatic individuals. *Am J Respir Crit Care Med* 158: 1487–1492

37   Shirakawa T, Mao X-Q, Sasaki S, Kawai M, Morimoto K, Hopkin JM (1996) Association between FcεRIβ and atopic disorders in a Japanese population. *Lancet* 347: 349–350

38   Palmer LJ, Pare PD, Faux JA, Moffatt MF, Daniels SE, LeSouf PN, Bremner PR, Mock-

ford E, Gracey M, Spargo R et al (1997) FcεRI-β polymorphism and total serum IgE levels in endemically parasitized Australian Aborigines. *Am J Hum Genet* 61: 182–188

39 Cox HE, Moffatt MF, Faux JA, Walley AJ, Coleman R, Trembath RC, Cookson WOCM, Harper JA (1998) Association of atopic dermatitis to the β subunit of the high affinity immunoglobulin E receptor. *Br J Dermatol* 138: 182–187

40 Tanaka K, Sugiura H, Uehara M, Sato H, Hashimoto-Tamaoki T, Furuyama J (1999) Association between mast cell chymase genotype and atopic eczema: comparison between patients with atopic eczema alone and those with atopic eczema and atopic respiratory disease. *Clin Exp Allergy* 29: 800–803

41 Hizawa N, Yamaguchi E, Jinushi E, Kawakami Y (2000) A common *FCER1B* promoter polymorphism influences total serum IgE levels in a Japanese population. *Am J Respir Crit Care Med* 161: 906–909

42 Kim Y-K, Ho S-H, Koh Y-Y, Son J-S, Lee B-J, Min K-M, Kim Y-Y (1999) Linkage between IgE receptor-mediated histamine releasability from basophils and gene marker of chromosome 11q13. *J Allergy Clin Immunol* 104: 618–622

43 Li A, Machay GA, Hopkin JM (1997) Functional analysis of histamine release from basophils and mast cells in subjects with Ile-181 to leu variant of FcεRIβ. *Clin Sci* 93: 279–286

44 Donnadeu E, Cookson WO, Jouvin M-H, Kinet J-P (2000) Allergy-associated polymorphisms of the FcεRIβ subunit do not impact its two amplification functions. *J Immunol* 165: 3917–3922

45 Lin S, Cicala C, Scharenberg AM, Kinet JP (1996) The FceRIb subunit functions as an amplifier of Fc(epsilon) RI gamma-mediated cell activation signals. *Cell* 85: 985–995

46 Hiraoka S, Furumoto Y, Koseki H, Takagaki Y, Taniguchi M, Okumura K, Ra C (1999) Fc receptor b subunit is requited for full activation of mast cells through Fc receptor engagement. *Int Immunol* 11: 199–207

47 Dombrowicz D, Lin S, Flammand V, Brini AT, Koller BH, Kinet J-P (1998) Allergy-associated FcεRIβ is a molecular amplifier of IgE- and IgG-medicated *in vivo* responses. *Immunity* 8: 517–529

48 Donnadeu E, Jouvin M-E, Kinet JP (2000) A second amplifier function for the allergy-associated FcεRIβ. *Immunity* 12: 515–523

49 Adra C, Lelias J-E, Kobayashi H, Kaghad M, Morrison P, Rowley JD, Lim B (1994) Cloning of the cDNA for a hematopoietic cell -specific protein related to CD20 and the β subunit of the high affinity IgE receptor : Evidence for a family of proteins with four transmembrane-spanning regions. *Proc Natl Acad Sci USA* 91: 10178–10182

50 Adra CN, Mao XQ, Kawada H, Gao PS, Korzycka B, Donate JL, Shaldon SR, Coull P, Dubowitz M, Enomoto T et al (1999) Chromosome 11q13 and atopic asthma. *Clin Genet* 55: 431–437

51 Beales PL, Warner AM, Hitman GA, Thakker R, Flinter FA (1997) Bardet-Biedl syndrome: a molecular and phenotypic study of 18 families. *J Med Genet* 34: 92–98

52 Laing IA, Goldblatt J, Eber E, Hayden CM, Rye PJ, Gibson NA, Palmer LJ, Burton PR,

LeSouf PN (1998) A polymorphism of the CC16 gene is associated with an increased risk of asthma. *J Med Genet* 35, 463–467

53   Gao P-S, Mao X-Q, Kawai M, Sasaki S, Tanabe O, Yoshimura K, Enomoto T, Shaldon SR, Dake Y, Kitano H et al (1998) Negative association between asthma and variants of CC16 in British and Japanese populations. *Hum Genet* 103: 57–59

54   Mao X-Q, Shirakawa T, Kawai M, Enomoto T, Sasaki S, Dake Y, Kitano H, Hagihara A, Hopkin JM, Morimoto K (1998) Association between asthma and an intragenic variant of CC16 on chromosome 11q13. *Clin Genet* 53: 54–56

55   Chapman CG, Browne J (1990) Isolation of the human ml(Hml) muscarinic acetylcholine receptor gene by PCR amplification. *Nucl Acid Res* 18: 2191

56   Neely JD, Buffy DL, Breazeale DR, Freidhoff LR, Schou C, Ehrlich-Kautzky E, Beaty T, Marsh DG (1996) Linkage analysis of IgE and chromosome 11q13. *Am J Respir Crit Care Med* 153: A767

57   Doull IJM, Lawrence S, Watson M, Begishvili T, Beasley RW, Lampe F, Holgate ST, Morton NE (1996) Allelic association of gene markers on chromosome 5q and 11q with atopy and bronchial hyperresponsiveness. *Am J Respir Crit Care Med* 153: 1280–1284

58   Hizawa N, Yamaguchi E, Furuya K, Ohnuma N, Kodama N, Kojima J, Ohe M, Kawakami Y (1995) Association between high serum total IgE levels and D11S97 on chromosome 11q13 in Japanese subjects. *J Med Genet* 32: 363–369

59   Wong ZY, Tsonls D, van Herwerden L, Raven J, Forbes A, Abramson MJ, Walter EH, Harrap SB (1997) Linkage analysis of bronchial hyperreactivity and atopy with chromosome 11q13. *Electrophoresis* 18: 1–5

60   CSGA (The collaborative study on the genetics of asthma) (1997) A genome-wide search for asthma susceptibility loci in ethnically diversed populations. *Nat Genet* 15: 389–392

Genetic regulation of interleukin-13 production

Tineke C.T.M. van der Pouw Kraan[1], John W. Holloway[2], Lucien A. Aarden[1] and Jaring S. van der Zee[3]

[1]Department of Molecular Cell Biology, VU Medical Center, Free University Amsterdam, The Netherlands; [2]Human Genetics Research Division, University of Southampton, Southampton General Hospital, Southampton, UK; [3]Department of Pulmonology, Academic Medical Center, Amsterdam, The Netherlands

Introduction

The 5q31-33 region contains a number of genes, including IL-13, that could be involved in the aetiology of allergic asthma. Other genes of interest in this region are the Th2 cytokines IL-4 and IL-5; the p40 chain of the Th1 cytokine inducer IL-12; IL-3; IL-9; CD14; the β_2-adrenergic receptor; the corticosteroid receptor and the transcription factors interferon regulatory factor 1 (IRF1) and transcription factor 7 (TCF7). Other diseases such as schistosomiasis may also be (at least partly) controlled by this region. In humans, the severity of infection caused by *Schistosoma mansoni* is linked to a marker on chromosome 5q31 [1]. In mice, resistance to this disease is regulated by Th2 cytokines; in particular, neutralisation of IL-13 leads to reduced pulmonary granuloma formation and total serum IgE levels, while Th2 cytokine production (IL-4, IL-5, and IL-13) remains intact [2]. The important role of Th2 cytokines in human asthma is underscored by the fact that T cells, acquired from bronchial biopsies, display an increased capacity to produce IL-4, IL-5, and IL-13 [3–5]. Interestingly, pulmonary expression of IL-13 is observed in both allergic and non-allergic asthma [6], while IL-4 expression may be more restricted to allergic asthma [7]. Because of their biological effects, IL-4 and IL-13, located at close proximity on 5q31, are very likely candidates to be involved in the inheritance of asthma. Firstly, for an antibody isotype switch to IgE, B cells require stimulation by either IL-4 or IL-13 [8, 9], and secondly these cytokines induce VCAM-1 expression on endothelial cells and pulmonary fibroblasts [10, 11], which may cause the accumulation of eosinophils at the site of the allergic reaction [12]. Recently, other effector functions of IL-4 and IL-13 have been described, independent of IgE and eosinophils.

The Hereditary Basis of Allergic Diseases, edited by Stephen T. Holgate and John W. Holloway
© 2002 Birkhäuser Verlag Basel/Switzerland

Animal studies

In mice, the control of Th2 responses is associated with a region on murine chromosome 11 that is syntenic with human chromosome 5q31 [13]. After the establishment of the critical role of Th2 cells in airway inflammation, the contribution of IL-4 was dissected. It turned out that Th2 cells from IL-4-deficient mice were inducing pulmonary mucus production as effectively as IL-4$^{+/+}$ Th2 cells [14]. The putative role of IL-13 in this process was confirmed later. Neutralisation of IL-13 during antigen challenge in sensitised mice leads to a reduction in airway hyperresponsiveness (AHR) and pulmonary mucus production [15, 16], independent of IgE and pulmonary eosinophilia. In contrast, neutralisation of IL-4 at this stage does not prevent pulmonary inflammation and AHR [17]. In addition, administration of IL-13 or IL-4 to non-immunised mice or selective expression of IL-13 in the lungs of IL-13-transgenic mice lead to the entire asthmatic phenotype [15, 16, 18]. Although IL-4 and IL-13 are both capable of inducing mucus production and airway hyper-responsiveness, IL-13 seems to be the critical cytokine during the effector stage of asthma. For the induction of Th2 responses, including IL-13 production, IL-4 may be the most important cytokine [19, 20]. The critical role of IL-13 in mucus production has also been observed in gastrointestinal nematode infection. While IL-4-deficient mice show a normal expulsion of *Nippostrongylus brasiliensis* [21], IL-13-deficient mice are no longer able to expel this nematode, despite a normal Th2 response [22]. This insufficiency is associated with a lack of mucus production in the gut. In this model, the activities of IL-4 and IL-13 are distinct and do not show redundancy. IL-13 appears to be the key cytokine for worm expulsion.

It has also become clear that the expression of the IL-4Rα is required for the effector function of IL-13. One of the events resulting from the triggering of the IL-4Rα is the activation of signal transducer and activator of transcription factor 6 (STAT-6). Neither IL-4 Rα- nor STAT-6-deficient mice are able to expel *N. brasiliensis* [23]. The same applies for the asthma models, while IL-4$^{-/-}$ Th2 cells are able to induce airway mucus formation and eosinophilia in normal mice, these cells failed to do so in IL-4Rα$^{-/-}$ mice [24], indicating that IL-13 requires IL-4Rα to exert its effects. In STAT-6-deficient mice, development of Th2 responses, AHR, IgE, and mucus production is abolished [25]. In both IL-4Rα$^{-/-}$ and STAT-6$^{-/-}$ mice, pulmonary eosinophilia and mucus production seem to be independent events, while only mucus production is dependent on IL-4Rα stimulation and subsequent STAT-6 activation.

IL-13 receptors

These overlapping but non-identical effects of IL-4 and IL-13 can be explained by the nature of the IL-13 receptor complexes. Initially, competitive binding studies on TF-1 cells, which respond to both IL-13 and IL-4, demonstrated that IL-13 can compete for the binding of IL-4 to its receptors and *vice versa*, suggesting that IL-4 receptor and IL-13 receptor complexes share a common component [26]. Subsequently, two IL-13-specific receptor subunits have been identified, IL-13 receptor α1 (IL-13Rα1) and α2 (IL-13Rα2).

IL-13Rα1 is a member of the haemopoetic receptor super family. Hilton et al. cloned the murine IL-13Rα1 on the basis of its conserved WSXWS motif and found that it has no homology with previously identified cytokine receptors [27]. By using transient expression of the mouse IL-13Rα1 cDNA in COS-7 cells, they found that it encodes a low affinity receptor capable of binding IL-13 but not IL-4 or other interleukins [27]. Subsequently, the human IL-13Rα1 was cloned by Aman et al. [28] and the gene was localised to the X chromosome.

In binding assays, minimal IL-13 binding activity is detected when 293T+ cells are transfected with IL-13Rα1. In contrast, co-expression of IL-4Rα results in significant binding of IL-13, indicating that IL-13Rα1 and IL-4Rα are shared components for IL-13 receptors [27]. Human IL-13Rα1 mRNA is expressed in multiple tissues including heart, liver, skeletal, muscle, ovary, brain, lung, and kidney by Northern blot [28].

The affinity of IL-13Rα1 for IL-13 is increased by the formation of a dimeric or trimeric receptor complex with the IL-4Rα chain and the γ_c subunit of the IL-4R (Type II and Type II IL-13 receptors) [29]. IL-13 or IL-4 binding to the IL-13Rα1/IL-4Rα receptor complex dimerises the receptor and activates the receptor-associated cytoplasmic tyrosine kinases, namely JAK-1 and Tyk-2. This leads to phosphorylation and activation of STAT-6 and STAT-3 as well as the IRS-1 and IRS-2 signalling pathways. This sharing of receptor components and signalling pathways accounts for the overlapping functions of IL-13 and IL-4.

Obiri et al. discovered that some human renal carcinoma cells (Caki-1 cells) express, in addition to receptors shared by IL-4 and IL-13, a large excess of specific IL-13 receptors [30]. Caput et al., after screening a panel of human carcinoma cell lines, first isolated cDNAs encoding the IL-13Rα2, a protein of 380 amino acids with a putative signal peptide of 26 amino acids, a single membrane-spanning domain, and a short cytoplasmic tail [31]. The IL-13Rα2 has homology with the human IL-5Rα chain (51% similarity and 27% identity).

Cells transfected with IL-13Rα2 show high ^{125}I-IL-13 binding that can be completely displaced by cold IL-13 but not by IL-4 [31]. Thus, IL-13Rα2 recognises IL-13 but not IL-4. However, COS cells expressing both IL-13Rα2 and IL-4Rα show similar binding for IL-13 to that of the cells expressing IL-13R alone, but 8–10% of that binding can be displaced by IL-4, suggesting the reconstitution of a binding site shared by both IL-13 and IL-4. The IL-13Rα2 gene has also been mapped to the X chromosome by Guo et al. [32]. It has been suggested that IL-13Rα2 is a decoy target for IL-13 and forms monomers that are non-signalling, with regard to STAT-6 activation and VCAM-1 induction [33]. Over-expression of IL-13Rα2 has been found in synovial cells, and it has been hypothesised that it can limit the function of

IL-13 in inflammatory joint disease [33]. The expression of IL-13Rα2 is extremely restricted; it is not expressed in peripheral blood mononuclear cells (PBMCs), and previously expression had been identified only in renal cell carcinoma cells, synovial cells, and glial cells. Using reverse transcriptase PCR (RT-PCR), we have shown high levels of expression of IL-13Rα2 on airway epithelium with lower levels of expression on bronchial fibroblasts (unpublished observations). As IL-13Rα2 binds IL-13 with higher affinity than IL-13Rα1 [34], this may be part of a compensatory mechanism limiting the function of IL-13 in the local tissue microenvironment. However, the function of IL-13Rα2 in normal or asthmatic bronchial epithelium or fibroblasts has not been investigated.

IL-13 and airway remodelling

In adults, only 50% of asthma is associated with atopy, yet all forms of the disease are characterised by enhanced T-cell secretion of Th2 cytokines in the airways. In addition, severe chronic asthma is characterised by the deposition of interstitial collagens in the *lamina reticularis* beneath the epithelial basement membrane associated with an increased number of myofibroblasts, epithelial damage, and increased mucus production airway remodelling [35, 36]. Of importance in asthma, IL-4 and IL-13 are key regulators of this response, with wide-ranging effects on epithelial cells, fibroblasts, and smooth muscle. As discussed above, the evidence suggesting a critical role for IL-13 in asthma comes from well-characterised experimental models of allergic asthma. Daily administration of IL-13 to the airways of mice has been shown to induce airway hyperresponsiveness, mucus secretion, goblet cell metaplasia, and subepithelial fibrosis [37, 38]. Similarly, transgenic expression of IL-13 in lung of mice has been shown to cause similar phenotypes [18].

In humans, treatment of bronchial epithelial cell with IL-13 leads to the secretion of TGF-α (which promotes mucus production), TGF-β_2 (profibrogenic), and inflammatory mediators such as IL-8 and GM-CSF (J. Lordan, D.E. Davies, personal communication). IL-13 induces expression of α-smooth muscle actin and a myofibroblast phenotype in primary lung fibroblasts [39] and acts on airway smooth muscle cells to alter responses to β-agonists [40].

Search for polymorphisms in the human IL-13 gene

For the IL-4 promoter and IL-4 receptor α chain, functional polymorphisms have been reported [41–44]. Because of the established importance of IL-13 in animal as well as human asthma, the hunt for polymorphisms in the IL-13 gene that could influence the asthmatic phenotype was started. Karen L. Anderson and colleagues analysed the IL-13 promoter region from −1039 to +80 in 129 individuals, comprising 96 patients with minimal-change nephropathy (which is associated with atopy) and 33 healthy people [45]. Single-strand conformation analysis indicated the absence of polymorphisms, a finding that made them doubt the significance of the IL-13 promoter as a susceptibility locus for atopy or any associated conditions. Marsha Wills-Karp and Lanny Rosenwasser confirmed these findings in the same report. After examination of the promoter region of IL-13 (the exact sequence examined was not mentioned) in a population of asthmatic families, no significant population-based promoter polymorphisms were found [45].

Aberrant T-cell IL-13 production in allergic asthma patients

We have examined the IL-13 promoter region based on our previous findings of the difference in regulation of IL-13 production by T cells from normal and allergic asthma individuals. We first examined the regulation of IL-13 production by T cells from normal individuals. Unexpectedly, a calcium-inducing signal was inhibitive for the production of IL-13 [46]. Differential stimulation of T cells allows determination of the magnitude of this negative signal: when T cells are stimulated with anti-CD28 and phorbol myristate acetate (PMA) (i.e., in the absence of a calcium signal), maximal IL-13 production is induced. Additional stimulation with anti-CD2, anti-CD3, or a calcium ionophore results in inhibition of IL-13 production on the protein as well as the mRNA level, which is reversed by cyclosporin A (CsA) (Fig. 1) ([46] and personal observations). We next compared the strength of this negative signal in T cells from allergic asthma with non-atopic controls. Interestingly, IL-13 production by T cells from allergic asthma patients is less sensitive for this inhibitory signal [47]. Because CsA prevents the calcium-induced inhibition of IL-13 production we speculated about the mechanism of this reduced inhibition of IL-13 production in allergic asthma patients. CsA is known to prevent the nuclear translocation of the transcription factor nuclear factor of activated T cells (NF-AT)p/c through inhibition of the calcium-dependent phosphatase calcineurin. In the absence of CsA, calcineurin activates NF-ATp/c by dephosphorylation [48], after which NF-AT translocates to the nucleus where it can bind to specific DNA sequences that control gene transcription. Therefore, a mutation in one of the consensus NF-AT sites of the IL-13 promoter could be an explanation for the observed difference between asthma patients and non-atopics in sensitivity of inhibition of IL-13 production by a calcium-inducing signal.

Identification of an IL-13 promoter polymorphism

Screening of the IL-13 promoter −1360 to −108 region by direct PCR sequencing, (allowing determination of both alleles simultaneously) led to the identification of

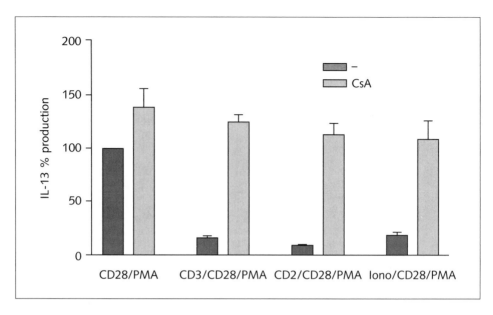

Figure 1

Inhibition of IL-13 production by a calcium-inducing stimulus is reversed by CsA. T cells from non-atopic individuals were activated by combinations of anti-CD28, PMA, anti-CD3, anti-CD2, and ionomycin as indicated. Supernatants were assayed for IL-13 production after a 3-day culture period. The mean results (± SE) of one representative experiment out of four are shown. (100% IL-13 production = 1761 pg/ml IL-13).

a nucleotide exchange (C to T) at position −1055, one nucleotide downstream of the consensus NF-AT site GGAAAA. In Figure 2, the −1055 genotypes of non-atopic controls and allergic asthma patients are compared with the percentage of maximal production of IL-13 (induced by anti-CD28 and PMA) after delivering the negative signal by anti-CD2. The −1055 TT genotype is associated with decreased relative inhibition of IL-13 production upon additional stimulation with anti-CD2, compared with the −1055 CC or −1055 CT genotypes ($p = 0.0016$ and $p = 0.0002$, respectively). This association was also apparent within the allergic asthma group: T cells from patients with the −1055 TT genotype were significantly less sensitive for the inhibitive signal ($p = 0.003$) compared with the remainder of these patients.

In addition, the −1055 TT genotype is associated with allergic asthma. In a case-control study, 101 allergic asthma patients and 107 non-atopic controls were screened for this IL-13 promoter polymorphism (Tab. 1). Allergic asthma patients show a higher frequency of the −1055 TT genotype (13/101 compared with 2/107 in the control group, $p = 0.002$, odds ratio $= 7.8$, RR $= 6.9$). The observation that the frequency of the −1055 TT genotype is higher in allergic asthma patients com-

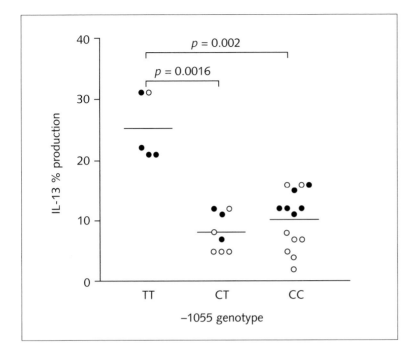

Figure 2
Association of the −1055 TT genotype with reduced inhibition of IL-13 production by anti-CD2. T cells from allergic asthma patients (•) and controls (○) were stimulated for 3 days with anti-CD28 and PMA, in the absence or presence of anti-CD2. The percentage production of IL-13 is shown after additional anti-CD2 stimulation is shown.

pared with non-atopic controls implies that this genotype could be associated with atopy, asthma, or both. However, we found no apparent correlation of the genotypes with total or specific serum IgE levels or BHR within the patient group.

From the animal studies mentioned above, it is clear that IL-13 is involved in mucus production. In human chronic obstructive pulmonary disease (COPD), extensive mucus hypersecretion is a prominent feature [49]. In our screening of pulmonary disease patients, we included eleven COPD patients; four of them were genotyped as −1055 TT (unpublished results). Compared with the frequency in non-atopic controls (2/107), the −1055 TT genotype is associated with COPD with an RR of 19 and an odds ratio of 30 ($p = 0.0006$). Although the frequency of −1055 TT carriers in COPD patients is not statistically different from the frequency in allergic asthma patients ($p = 0.06$), these data strongly suggest an important role for IL-13 in mucus production in human disease as well.

Table 1 - Association of the –1055 TT genotype with allergic asthma

–1055 genotype	allergic asthma patients n = 101	non-atopic controls n =107	
CC	57 (56%)	77 (72%)	$p = 0.02$
CT	31 (31%)	28 (26%)	
TT	13 (13%)	2 (2%)	$p = 0.002$

Patients and non-atopic controls were genotyped by sequencing and an IL-13 –1055-specific oligo-ligase-assay.

The IL-13 –1055 polymorphism influences binding of nuclear proteins

Analysis of the interaction between nuclear proteins from activated (anti-CD3/anti-CD28/PMA) peripheral blood T cells and this polymorphic region revealed a difference in binding pattern from the probes containing either T or C at position –1055. A high-molecular-weight complex was formed with the –1055-T sequence, but not with the –1055-C sequence (Fig. 3). These findings were confirmed in cross-competition experiments. We analysed the capacity of –1055 T and –1055 C and of an NF-AT sequence present in the IL-4 promoter to compete for binding of nuclear proteins to the –1055 T probe (Fig. 4). The high-molecular-weight complex was disrupted by unlabelled –1055 T, while –1055 C hardly affected binding of nuclear proteins to –1055 T. The IL-4 NF-AT sequence contains a T at the same position as the –1055-T sequence and also effectively competed for the high-molecular-weight complex, except for the upper band. These data indicate that the C- to T-change at position –1055 adjacent to the NF-AT site results in increased binding of nuclear proteins. The IL-4 NF-AT sequence, which did not compete for the upper band, indicates that the flanking region of the NF-AT site also influences binding of nuclear proteins. The nature of these proteins is currently unknown, but it is tempting to speculate that NF-AT family members are involved. Because CsA (which prevents NF-ATp/c translocation to the nucleus) upregulates IL-13 production, it is quite imaginable that binding of NF-AT to the promoter region of IL-13 reduces transcription. The –1055 TT genotype is associated with reduced sensitivity for inhibition by a CsA-sensitive signal. Therefore, it is logical to assume that the –1055 TT genotype would show decreased binding of nuclear proteins. However, the opposite is true. This puzzling phenomenon may be explained by studies performed in several NF-AT knockout mice. In NF-AT1- (= NF-ATp) or NF-AT4-deficient mice, an enhanced expression of IL-4 and IL-13 is observed [50–52]. In particular, the NF-AT1 and NF-AT4 double-deficient mice show a dramatic and specific

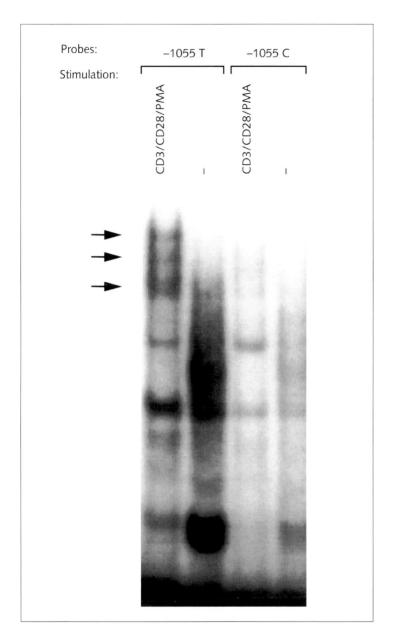

Figure 3
Increased binding of nuclear proteins to the −1055 T allele. ^{32}P-labelled probes of the −1055 T or −1055 C allele were incubated with nuclear extracts from unstimulated (−) or anti-CD3, anti-CD28 plus PMA-stimulated cells. The arrows indicate a high-molecular-weight complex selectively binding to the −1055 T sequence.

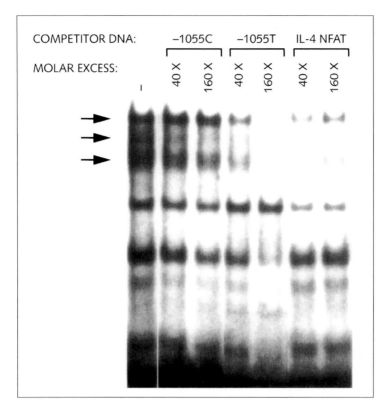

Figure 4
Cross competition of nuclear protein/-1055 T allele interactions. Nuclear extracts from acti-
vated T cells (anti-CD3, anti-CD28 and PMA) were incubated with ^{32}P-labelled –1055 T.
Protein DNA interactions were competed for by unlabelled –1055 T, –1055 C, or the NF-AT
sequence from the IL-4 promoter.

upregulation of Th2 cytokine expression. Interestingly, in these mice NF-ATc is present in large amounts in the nucleus [53], suggesting that NF-ATc positively affects Th2 cytokine production. In agreement with these results, NF-ATc- deficient mice have impaired Th2 responses [54, 55]. These studies indicate that NF-AT1 and NF-AT4 act as repressors of Th2 cytokine production, while NF-ATc is a positive regulator. The human IL-13 promoter contains three consensus NF-AT binding sites from which the net result may be a negative influence on IL-13 transcription. The C- to T-alteration at position –1055 may very well cause an increase in binding of nuclear proteins of NF-AT family members that positively influences IL-13 transcription.

Table 2 - Polymorphism of the IL-13 gene

Nucleotide position[a]	Position relative to +1 of ORF	Base change	location	Refs.
50012	−1512	A/C	promoter	[56]
49612	−1112[b]	C/T	promoter	[56, 59], this study
47959	−	G/C	Intron 1	[58]
46578	−	C/T	Intron 3	[56, 58]
46457	+389	G/A	Exon 4 (Arg110Gln)[c]	[56–58, 60]
45976	+870	G/A	Exon 4 (3'-UTR)	[56]
45921	+925	C/A	Exon 4 (3'-UTR)	[56, 58]
45752	+1094	C/T	Exon 4 (3'-UTR)	[56]

[a]*Genbank Accession Number AC004039;* [b]*position −1055 relative to transcription initiation site;* [c]*amino acid 131 in the pre-protein*

It cannot be ruled out that the IL-13 polymorphism is in fact linked to another polymorphism in the chromosome 5q31 region that influences the development of allergic asthma. However, because of the association of the −1055 TT genotype with altered regulation of IL-13 production and increase in nuclear protein binding, it is conceivable that the polymorphism itself is involved in the genetic susceptibility to allergic asthma.

Other polymorphisms of IL-13

Subsequent to the identification of the C-1055T promoter polymorphism of IL-13, several groups have screened the IL-13 gene for polymorphism [56–60]. A number of other polymorphisms were identified (Tab. 2). As well as additional promoter polymorphisms, an amino acid polymorphism of IL-13 has recently been identified, Arg110Gln [56–58, 60]. Protein modelling suggests that this polymorphism may influence binding of IL-13 to IL-4Rα [57]. The work of Graves et al. [56] and the more recent publication of Liu et al. [60] show strong associations between IL-13 polymorphisms and atopy in children. However, neither study examined associations with asthma. In contrast, the study of Heinzmann et al. [57] shows that, in a UK adult population, this polymorphism is associated with asthma, not atopy. The discrepancy in the association studies may be accounted for by the multiple roles IL-13 plays in allergic asthma, both in regulating IgE production and in driving airway remodelling in persistent disease. It is possible that polymorphisms in IL-13 may confer susceptibility to airway remodelling in asthma, as well as to allergic inflammation in early life.

Conclusions

The IL-4, IL-5, and IL-13 genes are closely linked, IL-4 and IL-13 being separated by only 12.5 kb, and IL-5 by 150 kb from IL-4 [61]. The gene complex is highly polymorphic, with both promoter and coding-region polymorphism potentially affecting the transcription and function of all three genes. In addition, all the transcription of IL-4, IL-13, and IL-5 is co-ordinately regulated as a single transcriptional unit. This occurs through long-range remodelling of the chromatin and concomitant increases in the accessibility of the genes to transcription factors [62] . Frazer et al. have identified several highly evolutionary conserved non-coding regions in the IL-4/IL-13 gene locus, including an 86 bp element located 5' of the IL-13 gene that is 91% identical to another non-coding element in the human 5q31 region, and a further 400 bp element located between the IL-4 and IL-13 genes (which is 85% identical in humans and mice). In human yeast artificial chromosome (YAC) transgenic mice lacking the 400 bp conserved element, production of human IL-4 and IL-13 is markedly reduced when compared with mice harbouring a wild-type YAC, strongly supporting its involvement in regulating the human IL-4 and IL-13 genes [63]. Thus, polymorphism outside of the immediate promoter and coding regions of IL-4 and IL-13 may also influence Th2 cytokine production and susceptibility to atopic disease.

In conclusion, it is apparent that there is a high degree of polymorphism of the IL-4/IL-13 gene locus and that this polymorphism may influence the development of Th2-type immune responses by individuals. This affects not only susceptibility of atopic disease but also response to parasitic infection and perhaps also modulates individuals' responses to Th1-dependant bacterial and viral infections. It is possible that polymorphism of IL-13 and elsewhere in the Th2 and Th1 ligand/receptor/signalling pathways has been conserved within the population by the selective influences of parasitic and bacterial/viral infections. Further research is needed to identify and type polymorphisms and extended haplotypes across the IL-4/IL-13 gene locus to distinguish true causative association from linkage disequilibrium, given the close proximity of the two genes. Further work is also needed to understand the effect of the different promoter haplotypes on gene transcription as well as the effects of the IL-13 R110Q polymorphism on receptor binding.

References

1   Marquet S, Abel L, Hillaire D, Dessein H, Kalil J, Feingold J, Weissenbach J, Dessein AJ (1996) Genetic localization of a locus controlling the intensity of infection by schistosoma mansoni on chromosome 5q31-q33. *Nat Genetics* 14: 181–184

2   Chiaramonte MG, Schopf LR, Neben TY, Cheever AW, Donaldson DD, Wynn TA (1999) IL-13 is a key regulatory cytokine for Th2 cell-mediated pulmonary granuloma formation and IgE responses induced by schistosoma mansoni eggs. *J Immunol* 162: 920–930

3   Del Prete GF, De Carli M, D'Elios MM, Maestrelli P, Ricci M, Fabbri L, Romagnani S (1993) Allergen exposure induces the activation of allergen-specific Th2 cells in the airway mucosa of patients with allergic respiratory disorders. *Eur J Immunol* 23: 1445–1449

4   Naseer T, Minshall EM, Leung DY, Laberge S, Ernst P, Martin RJ, Hamid Q (1997) Expression of IL-12 and IL-13 mRNA in asthma and their modulation in response to steroid therapy. *Am J Respir Crit Care Med* 155: 845–851

5   Robinson DS, Hamid Q, Ying S, Tsicopoulos A, Barkans J, Bentley AM, Corrigan C, Durham SR, Kay AB (1992) Predominant Th2-like bronchoalveolar T-lymphocyte population in atopic asthma. *N Engl J Med* 326: 298–304

6   Humbert M, Durham SR, Kimmitt P, Powell N, Assoufi B, Pfister R, Menz G, Kay AB, Corrigan CJ (1997) Elevated expression of messenger ribonucleic acid encoding IL-13 in the bronchial mucosa of atopic and nonatopic subjects with asthma. *J Allergy Clin Immunol* 99: 657–665

7   Walker C, Bode E, Boer L, Hansel TT, Blaser K, Virchow JC, Jr. (1992) Allergic and non-allergic asthmatics have distinct patterns of T-cell activation and cytokine production in peripheral blood and bronchoalveolar lavage. *Am Rev Respir Dis* 146: 109–115

8   Defrance T, Carayon P, Billian G, Guillemot JC, Minty A, Caput D, Ferrara P (1994) Interleukin 13 is a B cell stimulating factor. *J Exp Med* 179: 135–143

9   Punnonen J, Aversa G, Cocks BG, McKenzie AN, Menon S, Zurawski G, de Waal Malefyt R, de Vries JE (1993) Interleukin 13 induces interleukin 4-independent IgG4 and IgE synthesis and CD23 expression by human B cells. *Proc Natl Acad Sci USA* 90: 3730–3734

10 Bochner BS, Klunk DA, Sterbinsky SA, Coffman RL, Schleimer RP (1995) IL-13 selectively induces vascular cell adhesion molecule-1 expression in human endothelial cells. *J Immunol* 154: 799–803

11 Doucet C, Brouty-Boye D, Pottin-Clemenceau C, Jasmin C, Canonica GW, Azzarone B (1998) IL-4 and IL-13 specifically increase adhesion molecule and inflammatory cytokine expression in human lung fibroblasts. *Int Immunol* 10: 1421–1433

12 Ying S, Meng Q, Barata LT, Robinson DS, Durham SR, Kay AB (1997) Associations between IL-13 and IL-4 (mRNA and protein), vascular cell adhesion molecule-1 expression, and the infiltration of eosinophils, macrophages, and T cells in allergen-induced late-phase cutaneous reactions in atopic subjects. *J Immunol* 158: 5050–5057

13   Gorham JD, Guler ML, Steen RG, Mackey AJ, Daly MJ, Frederick K, Dietrich WF, Murphy KM (1996) Genetic mapping of a murine locus controlling development of T helper 1 T helper 2 type responses. *Proc Natl Acad Sci USA* 93: 12467–12472

14   Cohn L, Homer RJ, Marinov A, Rankin J, Bottomly K (1997) Induction of airway mucus production by T helper 2 (Th2) cells: A critical role for interleukin 4 in cell recruitment but not mucus production. *J Exp Med* 186: 1737–1747

15   Grunig G, Warnock M, Wakil AE, Venkayya R, Brombacher F, Rennick DM, Sheppard D, Mohrs M, Donaldson DD, Locksley RM et al (1998) Requirement for IL-13 independently of IL-4 in experimental asthma. *Science* 282: 2261–2263

16   Wills-Karp M, Luyimbazi J, Xu XY, Schofield B, Neben TY, Karp CL, Donaldson DD (1998) Interleukin-13: Central mediator of allergic asthma. *Science* 282: 2258–2261

17   Coyle AJ, Le Gros G, Bertrand C, Tsuyuki S, Heusser CH, Kopf M, Anderson GP (1995) Interleukin-4 is required for the induction of lung Th2 mucosal immunity. *Am J Respir Cell Mol Biol* 13: 54–59

18   Zhu Z, Homer RJ, Wang Z, Chen Q, Geba GP, Wang J, Zhang Y, Elias JA (1999) Pulmonary expression of interleukin-13 causes inflammation, mucus hypersecretion, subepithelial fibrosis, physiologic abnormalities, and eotaxin production. *J Clin Invest* 103: 779–788

19   Sornasse T, Larenas PV, Davis KA, de Vries JE, Yssel H (1996) Differentiation and stability of T helper 1 and 2 cells derived from naive human neonatal CD4[+] T cells, analyzed at the single-cell level. *J Exp Med* 184: 473–483

20   Zurawski G, de Vries JE (1994) Interleukin 13, an interleukin 4-like cytokine that acts on monocytes and B cells, but not on T cells. *Immunol Today* 15: 19–26

21   Lawrence RA, Gray CA, Osborne J, Maizels RM (1996) Nippostrongylus brasiliensis: Cytokine responses and nematode expulsion in normal and IL-4-deficient mice. *Exp Parasitol* 84: 65–73

22   McKenzie GJ, Bancroft A, Grencis RK, McKenzie ANJ (1998) A distinct role for interleukin-13 in Th2-cell-mediated immune responses. *Current Biology* 8: 339–342

23   Urban JF Jr, Noben-Trauth N, Donaldson DD, Madden KB, Morris SC, Collins M, Finkelman FD (1998) IL-13, IL-4Ralpha, and stat6 are required for the expulsion of the gastrointestinal nematode parasite nippostrongylus brasiliensis. *Immunity* 8: 255–264

24   Cohn L, Homer RJ, MacLeod H, Mohrs M, Brombacher F, Bottomly K (1999) Th2-induced airway mucus production is dependent on IL-4Ralpha, but not on eosinophils. *J Immunol* 162: 6178–6183

25   Kuperman D, Schofield B, Wills-Karp M, Grusby MJ (1998) Signal transducer and activator of transcription factor 6 (stat6)-deficient mice are protected from antigen-induced airway hyperresponsiveness and mucus production. *J Exp Med* 187: 939–948

26   Obiri NI, Leland P, Murata T, Debinski W, Puri RK (1997) The IL-13 receptor structure differs on various cell types and may share more than one component with IL-4 receptor. *J Immunol* 158: 756–764

27   Hilton DJ, Zhang JG, Metcalf D, Alexander WS, Nicola NA, Willson TA (1996)

Cloning and characterization of a binding subunit of the interleukin 13 receptor that is also a component of the interleukin 4 receptor. *Proc Natl Acad Sci USA* 93: 497–501

28   Aman MJ, Tayebi N, Obiri NI, Puri RK, Modi WS, Leonard WJ (1996) cDNA cloning and characterization of the human interleukin 13 receptor alpha chain. *J Biol Chem* 271: 29265–29270

29   Murata T, Taguchi J, Puri RK, Mohri H (1999) Sharing of receptor subunits and signal transduction pathway between the IL-4 and IL-13 receptor system. *Int J Hematol* 69: 13–20

30   Obiri NI, Debinski W, Leonard WJ, Puri RK (1995) Receptor for interleukin 13. Interaction with interleukin 4 by a mechanism that does not involve the common gamma chain shared by receptors for interleukins 2, 4, 7, 9, and 15. *J Biol Chem* 270: 8797–8804

31   Caput D, Laurent P, Kaghad M, Lelias JM, Lefort S, Vita N, Ferrara P (1996) Cloning and characterization of a specific interleukin (IL)-13 binding protein structurally related to the IL-5 receptor alpha chain. *J Biol Chem* 271: 16921–16926

32   Guo JA, Apiou F, Mellerin MP, Lebeau B, Jacques Y, Minvielle S (1997) Chromosome mapping and expression of the human interleukin-13 receptor. *Genomics* 42: 141–145

33   Feng NP, Lugli SM, Schnyder B, Gauchat JFM, Graber P, Schlagenhauf E, Schnarr B, Wiederkehr-Adam M, Duschl A, Heim MH et al (1998) The interleukin-4/interleukin-13 receptor of human synovial fibroblasts: Overexpression of the nonsignaling interleukin-13 receptor alpha 2. *Lab Invest* 78: 591–602

34   Donaldson DD, Whitters MJ, Fitz LJ, Neben TY, Finnerty H, Henderson SL, O'Hara RM, Beier DR, Turner KJ, Wood CR et al (1998) The murine IL-13 receptor alpha 2: Molecular cloning, characterization, and comparison with murine IL-13 receptor alpha 1. *J Immunol* 161: 2317–2324

35   Elias JA, Zhu Z, Chupp G, Homer RJ (1999) Airway remodeling in asthma. *J Clin Invest* 104: 1001–1006

36   Holgate ST, Lackie PM, Howarth PH, Roche WR, Puddicombe SM, Richter A, Wilson SJ, Holloway JW, Davies DE (2001) Activation of the epithelial mesenchymal trophic unit in the pathogenesis of asthma. *Int Arch Allergy Immunol* 124: 253–258

37   Grunig G, Warnock M, Wakil AE, Venkayya R, Brombacher F, Rennick DM, Sheppard D, Mohrs M, Donaldson DD, Locksley RM et al (1998) Requirement for IL-13 independently of IL-4 in experimental asthma. *Science* 282: 2261–2263

38   Wills-Karp M, Luyimbazi J, Xu X, Schofield B, Neben TY, Karp CL, Donaldson DD (1998) Interleukin-13: Central mediator of allergic asthma. *Science* 282: 2258–2261

39   Hashimoto S, Gon Y, Takeshita I, Maruoka S, Horie T (2001) IL-4 and IL-13 induce myofibroblastic phenotype of human lung fibroblasts through c-jun NH2-terminal kinase-dependent pathway. *J Allergy Clin Immunol* 107: 1001–1008

40   Laporte JC, Moore PE, Baraldo S, Jouvin MH, Church TL, Schwartzman IN, Panettieri RA Jr, Kinet JP, Shore SA (2001) Direct effects of interleukin-13 on signaling pathways for physiological responses in cultured human airway smooth muscle cells. *Am J Respir Crit Care Med* 164: 141–148

41 Deichmann K, Bardutzky J, Forster J, Heinzmann A, Kuehr J (1997) Common poly-morphisms in the coding part of the IL4-receptor gene. *Biochem Biophys Res Comm* 231: 696–697

42 Hershey GKK, Friedrich MF, Esswein LA, Thomas ML, Chatila TA (1997) The associ-ation of atopy with a gain-of-function mutation in the alpha subunit of the interleukin-4 receptor. *N Engl J Med* 337: 1720–1725

43 Mitsuyasu H, Izuhara K, Mao XQ, Gao PS, Arinobu Y, Enomoto T, Kawai M, Sasaki S, Dake Y, Hamasaki N et al (1998) Ile50val variant of IL4Ra upregulates IgE synthe-sis and associates with atopic asthma. *Nat Genetics* 19: 119–120

44 Rosenwasser LJ, Klemm DJ, Dresback JK, Inamura H, Mascali JJ, Klinnert M, Borish L (1995) Promoter polymorphisms in the chromosome 5 gene cluster in asthma and atopy. *Clin Exp Allergy* 25: 74–78

45 Anderson K, Mathieson P, Gillespie K (1999) Polymorphisms not found in the IL-13 gene promoter. *Science* 284: 1431

46 van der Pouw Kraan TC, Boeije LC, Troon JT, Rutschmann SK, Wijdenes J, Aarden LA (1996) Human IL-13 production is negatively influenced by CD3 engagement. Enhance-ment of IL-13 production by cyclosporin a. *J Immunol* 156: 1818–1823

47 van der Pouw Kraan T, Van der Zee JS, Boeije LCM, De Groot ER, Stapel SO, Aarden LA (1998) The role of IL-13 in IgE synthesis by allergic asthma patients. *Clin Exp Immunol* 11: 129–135

48 Rao A (1994) NF-ATp: A transcription factor required for the co-ordinate induction of several cytokine genes. *Immunol Today* 15: 274–281

49 Jeffery PK (1999) Differences and similarities between chronic obstructive pulmonary disease and asthma. *Clin Exp Allergy* 29 (Suppl 2): 14–26

50 Hodge MR, Ranger AM, Charles de la Brousse F, Hoey T, Grusby MJ, Glimcher LH (1996) Hyperproliferation and dysregulation of IL-4 expression in NF-ATp-deficient mice. *Immunity* 4: 397–405

51 Kiani A, Viola JP, Lichtman AH, Rao A (1997) Down-regulation of IL-4 gene tran-scription and control of Th2 cell differentiation by a mechanism involving NFAT1. *Immunity* 7: 849–860

52 Viola JP, Kiani A, Bozza PT, Rao A (1998) Regulation of allergic inflammation and eosinophil recruitment in mice lacking the transcription factor NFAT1: Role of inter-leukin-4 (IL-4) and IL-5. *Blood* 91: 2223–2230

53 Ranger AM, Oukka M, Rengarajan J, Glimcher LH (1998) Inhibitory function of two NFAT family members in lymphoid homeostasis and Th2 development. *Immunity* 9: 627–635

54 Ranger AM, Hodge MR, Gravallese EM, Oukka M, Davidson L, Alt FW, de la Brousse FC, Hoey T, Grusby M, Glimcher LH (1998) Delayed lymphoid repopulation with defects in IL-4-driven responses produced by inactivation of NF-ATc. *Immunity* 8: 125–134

55 Yoshida H, Nishina H, Takimoto H, Marengere LE, Wakeham AC, Bouchard D, Kong

YY, Ohteki T, Shahinian A, Bachmann M et al (1998) The transcription factor NF-ATc1 regulates lymphocyte proliferation and Th2 cytokine production. *Immunity* 8: 115–124

56 Graves PE, Kabesch M, Halonen M, Holberg CJ, Baldini M, Fritzsch C, Weiland SK, Erickson RP, von Mutius E, Martinez FD (2000) A cluster of seven tightly linked polymorphisms in the IL-13 gene is associated with total serum IgE levels in three populations of white children. *J Allergy Clin Immunol* 105: 506–513

57 Heinzmann A, Mao X-Q, Akaiwa M, Kreomer RT, Gao P-S, Oshima K, Umeshita R, Abe Y, Braun S, Yamashita T et al (2000) Genetic variants of IL-13 signalling and human asthma and atopy. *Hum Mol Genetics* 9: 549–559

58 Pantelidis P, Jones MG, Welsh KI, Taylor AN, du Bois RM (2000) Identification of four novel interleukin-13 gene polymorphisms. *Genes Immun* 1: 341–345

59 Laundy GJ, Spink CF, Keen LJ, Wood NA, Bidwell JL (2000) A novel polymorphism in the human interleukin-13 (IL-13) promoter. *Eur J Immunogenetics* 27: 53–54

60 Liu X, Nickel R, Beyer K, Wahn U, Ehrlich E, Freidhoff LR, Bjorksten B, Beaty TH, Huang SK (2000) An IL13 coding region variant is associated with a high total serum IgE level and atopic dermatitis in the german multicenter atopy study (mas-90). *J Allergy Clin Immunol* 106: 167–170

61 Frazer KA, Ueda Y, Zhu Y, Gifford VR, Garofalo MR, Mohandas N, Martin CH, Palazzolo MJ, Cheng JF, Rubin EM (1997) Computational and biological analysis of 680 kb of DNA sequence from the human 5q31 cytokine gene cluster region. *Genome Research* 7: 495–512

62 Agarwal S, Rao A (1998) Modulation of chromatin structure regulates cytokine gene expression during T cell differentiation. *Immunity* 9: 765–775

63 Loots GG, Locksley RM, Blankespoor CM, Wang ZE, Miller W, Rubin EM, Frazer KA (2000) Identification of a coordinate regulator of interleukins 4, 13, and 5 by cross-species sequence comparisons. *Science* 288: 136–140

The role of interleukin-9 and the interleukin-9 receptor gene candidates in asthma

Roy C. Levitt, Michael P. McLane, Luigi Grasso and Nicholas C. Nicolaides

Genaera Institute of Molecular Medicine, Genarea Corporation, Plymouth Meeting, 5110 Campus Drive, Plymouth Meeting, PA 19462, USA

Introduction

It is now generally well accepted that atopic asthma is a complex heritable disorder of the airways in which symptoms depend on environmental exposure [1]. This lung disorder is associated with clinical signs and symptoms of airway hyperresponsiveness (AHR), an exaggerated narrowing of the airways to provocative stimuli, and eosinophilic inflammation associated with reversible airway obstruction. Significant biologic variability in airway responsiveness occurs in humans, and baseline bronchial hyperresponsiveness is recognized as a heritable risk factor for asthma [2–5]. While significant biologic variability in airway responsiveness in rodents and humans has been observed, little is understood about the genetic regulation of AHR [5]. Moreover, it remains unclear whether or how AHR is associated with an underlying predisposition to eosinophilic airway inflammation. Recently, genetic linkage studies and functional genomics in humans and mice have implicated interleukin-9 (IL-9) and its receptor in the genetics of AHR and asthma [6–15]. In this chapter, we will review evidence supporting a central role for IL-9 as a regulator of AHR and a critical mediator of allergic asthma and mucosal Th2 immunity.

Genetic analysis of AHR identifies the IL-9 gene candidate

Chromosome 5q31-q33 is one location where asthma and its risk factors have previously been mapped by genetic linkage, including elevated serum IgE and AHR [6–8, 10, 11]. Linkage studies in mice pinpointed a smaller region on chromosome 13 associated with AHR in conservation with this much larger segment of chromosome 5q in humans (Fig. 1) [9]. Analyses of murine gene candidates on chromosome

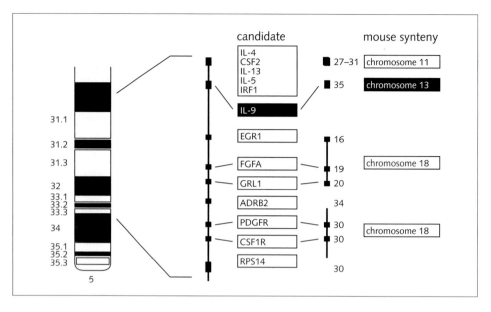

Figure 1

Random genetic analyses identifies IL-9 asthma gene candidate.

Illustration of the genetic map of human chromosome 5q31-q33 and syntenic regions in the mouse. The region of human chromosome 5q31-q33 demonstrating evidence for linkage with AHR is homologous to portions of mouse chromosomes 11, 13, and 18. Chromosome 13 contains the IL-9 gene candidate and was linked to baseline AHR in mouse and man. Data are from [9]. Figure reproduced with permission from the publisher of PNAS.

13 identified a genetic defect at the C57BL/6 (B6) IL-9 locus associated with no detectable lung IL-9 expression and reduced airway responsiveness in naïve B6 mice (Fig. 2). In contrast, robust levels of lung IL-9 were observed in DBA/2J mice associated with AHR. Furthermore, (B6D2)F1 mice were intermediate in airway responsiveness and lung IL-9 levels, demonstrating a tight genotype-phenotype relation (Fig. 2). These same inbred strains did not differ in lung levels of IL-4, IL-5, or IL-13. Human studies further corroborate these animal data. Lung IL-9 levels as determined by immunocytochemistry and *in situ* hybridization demonstrate a highly significant and specific association between the expression of this cytokine with asthma and airway hyperresponsiveness to methacholine [16]. In contrast, IL-9 levels in bronchial biopsies from patients with chronic bronchitis, sarcoidosis, atopic allergy (without asthma), and normal lung status were not associated with elevated IL-9 levels [16] (Fig. 3). Thus, biologic variability in lung IL-9 levels appeared to be determined genetically, and high lung levels of this cytokine in humans are tightly and specifically associated with AHR and asthma.

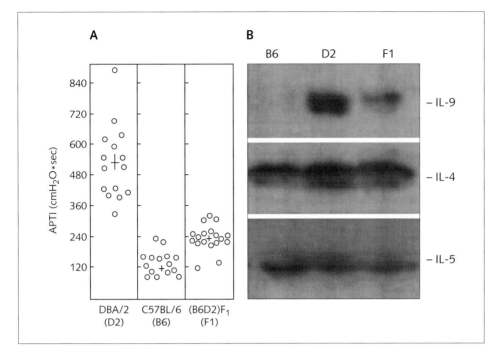

Figure 2
Genetic defect at IL-9 locus effects expression and AHR in mice.
A strong genotype-phenotype relation is demonstrated between airway responsiveness and lung IL-9 levels in the DBA/2 (D2), C57BL/6 (B6), and (C57BL/6 X DBA/2)F1 (F1) mice. (A) Airway pressure time index (APTI) [9] response to a bronchochonstrictor is shown for individual D2, B6, and F1 animals. This quantitative trait was mapped to a QTL on murine chromosome 13 (see Fig. 1). (B) Western blot analysis of cytokines from the lungs of hyporesponsive B6, hyperresponsive D2, and intermediate responding F1 inbred mice. This blot demonstrates reduced steady-state lung IL-9 protein level at baseline in naïve B6 mice, compared with intermediate levels in F1 mice, and robust levels in D2 mice. Data are from [9]. Figure reproduced with permission from the publisher of PNAS.

Established functions of IL-9 consistent with its role in asthma

Our linkage studies searched randomly for any genes involved in murine AHR that corresponded to the region linked to asthma phenotypes on human chromosome 5q. A quantitative trait locus (QTL) on murine chromosome 13 prompted us to examine the IL-9 candidate (Fig. 1) [9]. While little was understood about this cytokine's role in asthma initially, a pleiotropic role for IL-9 in the allergic response is now

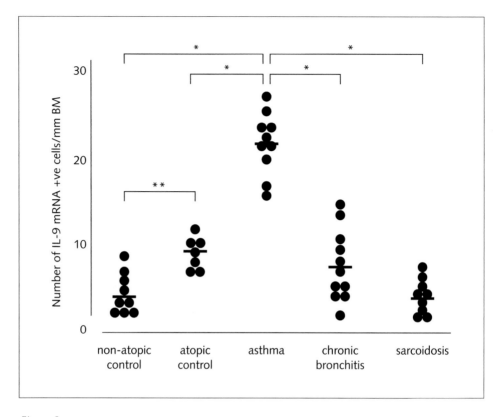

Figure 3
Increased expression of lung IL-9 transcript and protein in subjects with atopic allergy and asthma.

IL-9 mRNA expression lung biopsies from nonatopic controls, atopic subjects without asthma, atopic asthmatics, chronic bronchitics, and subjects with sarcoidosis. Results are expressed as numbers of positive cells per millimeter of basement membrane. IL-9 expression was increased significantly in asthmatics as compared with all other subjects (P < 0.001). IL-9 expression was increased to a lesser degree in atopic subjects as compared with non-atopic controls (P < 0.05). Similar results were observed when IL-9 immunoreactive cells were examined in these subjects. All data are from [16]. Figure reproduced with permission from the publisher of J. Allergy Clin. Immunol.

supported by numerous independent studies [17–24]. IL-9 is a T-cell growth factor, and experimental data have shown a correlation between IL-9 production and Th2-responses *in vivo* [17]. IL-9 was originally described as a mast cell growth factor and likely impacts IgE-mediated responses by upregulating the expression of the alpha chain of the high-affinity IgE receptor, and mast cell mediators [18, 19]. In addition, *in vitro* and *in vivo* studies have shown IL-9 to potentiate the release of IgE from primed B cells, which is considered to be a hallmark of atopic allergy and a risk factor for asthma [20, 21]. IL-9 promotes eosinophilic inflammation by stimulating the production of a number of chemokines including eotaxin, MCP1, MCP3, MCP5, MIP1α, and MIP1β [22]. The upregulation of IL-5Rα by IL-9 likely impacts downstream, IL-5-mediated features of the allergic inflammatory response [23].

IL-9 transgenic animals have increased responsiveness to antigen and an asthmatic phenotype

Two independent IL-9 transgenic models have also been developed [14, 15]. Naïve IL-9 transgenic mice resemble allergic asthma including AHR, eosinophilia, mucus hypersecretion, increased serum total IgE, and mast cell hyperplasia with intraepithelial mast cells [15]. The MUC2 and MUC5AC gene products appear to be specifically associated with the gross over-production of mucus in IL-9 transgenic mice [24]. Importantly, antigen-driven inflammation was also significantly upregulated in IL-9 transgenic mice compared with genetic controls (FVB/N background strain), suggesting a role for this cytokine in regulating mucosal Th2 immunity and asthma [14] (Fig. 4). Mast cells are important effector cells in asthma, and increased lung mast cell numbers have not been observed commonly in murine allergic inflammatory models associated with other Th2 cytokines. In contrast, increased numbers of intra-epithelial lung mast cells were a noteworthy finding in both of these IL-9 transgenic models [14, 15].

Lung instillation of recombinant IL-9 (rIL-9) in B6 mice produces an asthmatic phenotype

To further evaluate *in vivo* whether IL-9 is sufficient to promote the pathophysiology of asthma, we instilled rIL-9 into the airways of B6 mice, previously shown to be genetically deficient in lung IL-9 protein [9, 23, 24]. After 10 days of intra-tracheal rIL-9 administration, levels of IL-9 were significantly increased on Western blot in the airways of B6 mice [23]. Lung instillation of rIL-9 produced all of the histopathologic features of asthma. These findings included a time- and dose dependent increase in the number of bronchoalveolar lavage (BAL) eosinophils, increased mucin and IL-5Rα gene expression (Figs. 5A and 5B), elevations in mean serum total IgE [9, 23, 24], and the induction of lung proteases along with submucosal membrane thickening (unpublished observations). Consistent with observations in IL-9 transgenic animals, the significant increase by IL-9 of mucus production was associated with the specific upregulation of MUC2 and MUC5AC mucin gene prod-

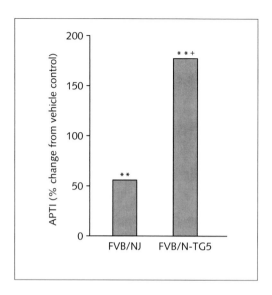

Figure 4

IL-9 promotes antigen-induced inflammation and AHR in transgenic mice.
*Airway response (APTI) to 5-HT after antigen exposure in FVB/NJ and FVB/N-TG5 mice is plotted as percent change from vehicle control animals. The antigen-induced airway respon-siveness of the FVB/N-TG5 mice was significantly greater than the response of identically treated FVB/NJ mice. Number of antigen-treated mice equals 15–19/strain. Analyses were run as a two-way ANOVA with subsequent comparisons by Bonferroni's t-test. The overall statistical analysis showed a group-wise treatment interaction (F = 13.54; P < 0.001). Sym-bols: ** denotes significantly different from same-strain vehicle-treated mice at P < 0.01 level, denotes significantly different from FVB/NJ mice (same treatment) at P < 0.05 level. Data are from [14]. Figure reproduced with permission from the publisher of AJRCMB.*

ucts [24]. These data further suggest that IL-9 is sufficient to produce a classical Th2 response *in vivo* and regulates baseline AHR and serum total IgE. Moreover, ampli-fication of mucosal antigen responses in the IL-9 transgenic relative to the controls suggests that IL-9 is a critical factor in mucosal Th2 immunity.

IL-9 neutralizing antibody ablates the asthmatic response in a model of mucosal Th2 immunity to natural antigens

Mice were sensitized and challenged intra-nasally with natural allergens without adjuvant in an established model of Th2 mucosal immunity that simulates asthma

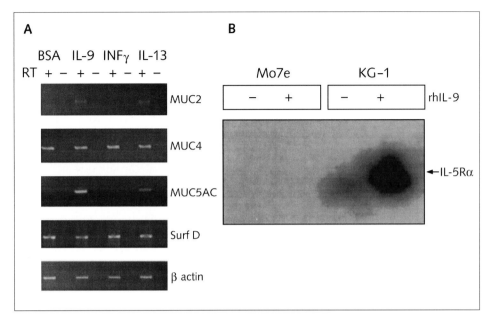

Figure 5
IL-9 directly upregulates the expression of IL-5Rα and specific mucins.
IL-9 has a direct effect on cells implicated in the pathophysiology of asthma. IL-9 stimulates IL-5Rα in purified cell populations and mucin expression and production in airway epithelial cells both in vitro and in vivo. (A) MUC2 and MUC5AC genes are induced in the whole lung of B6 mice when rIL-9 is instilled into the airways. In contrast, BSA carrier or recombinant interferon gamma does not have a similar effect [24]. Briefly, recombinant cytokines with BSA carrier were instilled into the lungs of mice, and whole lung tissues were analyzed for expression of mucin and control transcripts by RT-PCR. Reverse transcriptase was withheld in (–) lanes and added in lanes marked by a (+). Data are from [24]. Figure reproduced with permission from publisher of AJRCMB. (B) IL-9 stimulates the expression of IL-5Rα specifically in eosinophil precursors. Data are from [23]. Figure reproduced with permission from the publisher of J. Allergy Clin. Immunol.

[14, 25]. Dust-mite antigen (DMA) produced a significant allergic inflammatory response in (B6D2)F1 [25]. This method produced sensitization and a complete constellation of allergic inflammatory responses including significant increases in BAL eosinophils, elevated serum total IgE, and AHR as compared with control or naïve animals. Overall histopathologic grade was significantly greater for DMA-treated animals as compared with control or naïve animals. Inflammatory cells were noted primarily in perivascular spaces, with minimal infiltration of alveolar air-spaces. In

addition, increased mucin production was also observed after PAS staining by histologic grading [25].

To determine whether IL-9 is a necessary mediator of Th2 mucosal immunity, IL-9 neutralizing antibody was instilled directly into the lungs of mice exposed to DMA in this asthma model of mucosal Th2 immunity [25]. Intra-tracheal administration of neutralizing antibody significantly reduced the complete constellation of allergic inflammatory findings in this model [25]. AHR, serum total IgE elevations, and increases in BAL eosinophils were reduced in comparison to isotype-specific control antibody. Mucin staining and overall histopathologic grading confirmed that the antibody treatment effectively abrogated the allergic asthmatic response in the antigen-challenged animals. DMA-specific serum IgG1 levels confirmed that these animals were sensitized to allergen by the methods employed (unpublished data). Collectively, these data demonstrate that IL-9 is both necessary and sufficient to produce the asthmatic response. In particular, IL-9 represents a critical factor in mucosal Th2 immunity and regulates the asthma risk factors AHR and elevated serum IgE. Thus, IL-9 represents an important therapeutic target in asthma.

Genetic analysis of asthma and AHR identifies the IL-9R gene candidate

Based on data establishing IL-9 as an asthma gene candidate, we examined the long arm XY pseudo-autosomal region for linkage to asthma, serum IgE, and bronchial hyperresponsiveness. Physical mapping studies suggest that this genomic region is approximately 320 kb in size and contains the IL-9 receptor gene [12, 26]. Multipoint non-parametric analyses provide evidence for linkage between DXYS154 and bronchial hyperresponsiveness (P = 0.000057) or asthma (P = 0.00065) [12] (Fig. 6). These results are consistent with the localization of a major gene controlling asthma and AHR to this small unique region of the genome and implicate the IL-9R as a potential asthma-gene candidate. Further molecular analyses of IL-9R transcripts identified multiple expressed variants, one of which is unable to bind IL-9 and may be involved in the down regulation of IL-9 activity *in vivo* [13].

Conclusions

Here we have reviewed genetic, physiologic, and functional studies that identify IL-9 and its receptor as key mediators of atopic asthma as diagrammed in Figure 7. In this chapter we have demonstrated that IL-9 is both necessary and sufficient to produce all of the histopathologic features of allergic asthma in mice. Importantly, IL-9-specific blockade ablated the asthma phenotype after mucosal antigen sensitization. These data are consistent with a critical role for IL-9 in antigen-driven mucos-

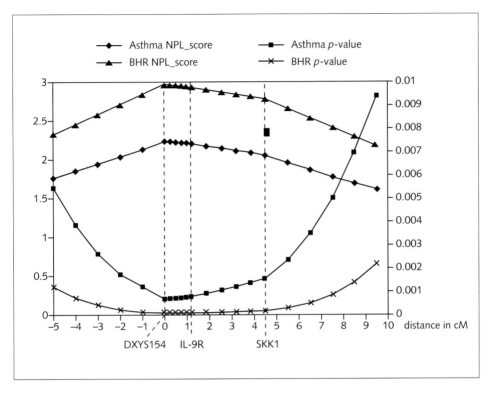

Figure 6
Mapping of asthma traits to the IL9R region of the XqYq chromosomes.
Multipoint three-locus linkage map localizing asthma traits in the genetic map of the XqYq
pseudo-autosomal region. Shown along the x axis is the most likely sex-averaged map of the
three genetic markers localized to the region. Plotted on the y axis are the multipoint MPL
scores for the asthma (diamonds) and AHR (triangles) phenotypes at various locations with
the map. Plotted on the secondary y axis are the exact P values (generated by GENEHUNTER)
on a log scale for the corresponding NPL scores (asthma, squares; AHR, x). Data are from
[12]. Figure reproduced with permission from the publisher of Genomics.

al Th2 immunity. Moreover, taking into account data on the classical pathways described for Th2 immunity, our data are consistent with either multiple parallel pathways or the classical pathways described for Th2 immunity lying downstream of IL-9/IL-9R actions. Nevertheless, this pathway may underlie in humans the genetic associations between asthma and chromosomes 5q31-q33, where the IL-9 locus is mapped, and the XY chromosome pseudo-autosomal region, where the IL-9 receptor is located.

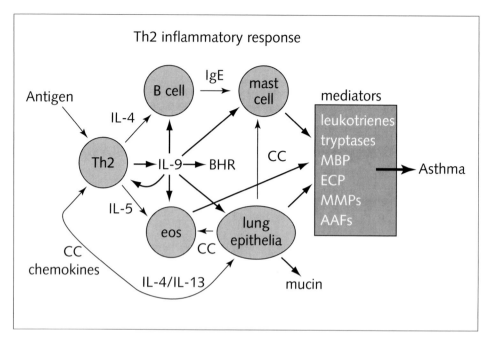

Figure 7

From antigen to asthma: IL-9 as a central regulator of Th2 inflammatory response. Antigen presentation to Th2 lymphocytes induces the release of IL-9. IL-9 induces mast cells, lung epithelia, eosinophils, B cells and Th2 lymphocytes to release a variety of cytokines, chemokines, IgE, mucus, and inflammatory mediators in a pathogenic sequelae that results in asthma.

References

1 Holgate ST, Church MK, Howarth PH, Morton NE, Frew AJ, Ratko D (1995) Genetic and environmental influences on airway inflammation in asthma. *Int Arch Allergy Immunol* 107: 29–33

2 Townley RG, Bewtra AK, Wilson AF, Hopp RJ, Elston RC, Nair NM, Watt GD (1986) Segregation analysis of bronchial response to methacholine inhalation challenge in families with and without asthma. *J Allergy Clin Immunol* 77: 101–107

3 Hopp RJ, Bewtra AK, Biven R, Nair NM, Townley RG (1988) Bronchial reactivity pattern in nonasthmatic parents of asthmatics. *Ann Allergy* 61: 184–186

4 Hopp RJ, Townley RG, Biven RE, Bewtra AK, Nair NM (1990) The presence of airway reactivity before the development of asthma. *Am Rev Respir Dis* 141: 2–8

5 Levitt RC, Mitzner W, Kleeberger SR (1990) A genetic approach to the study of lung

physiology: understanding biological variability in airway responsiveness. *Am J Physiol* 258 (4 Pt 1): L157–L164

6   Meyers DA, Postma DS, Panhuysen CI, Xu J, Amelung PJ, Levitt RC, Bleecker ER (1994) Evidence for a locus regulating total serum IgE levels mapping to chromosome 5. *Genomics* 23 (2): 464–470

7   Marsh DG, Neely JD, Breazeale DR, Ghosh B, Freidhoff LR, Ehrlich-Kautzky E, Schou C, Krishnaswamy G, Beaty TH (1994) Linkage analysis of IL4 and other chromosome 5q311 markers and total serum immunoglobulin E concentrations. *Science* 264: 1152–1156

8   Postma DS, Beecker ER, Amelung PJ, Holroyd KJ, Xu J, Panhuysen CIM, Meyers DA, Levitt RC (1995) Genetic susceptibility to asthma – bronchial hyperresponsiveness coinherited with a major gene for atopy. *N Engl J Med* 333: 894–900

9   Nicolaides NC, Holroyd KC, Ewart SL, Eleff SM, Kiser MB, Dragwa CR, Sullivan CD, Grasso L, Zhang LY, Messler CJ et al (1997) Interleukin-9: A candidate gene for asthma. *Proc Natl Acad Sci USA* 94: 13175–13180

10 Doull I, Lawrence S, Watson M, Begishvili T, Beasley R, Lampe F, Holgate ST, Morton NE (1996) Allelic association of gene markers on chromosomes 5q and 11q with atopy and bronchial hyperresponsiveness. *Am J Respir Crit Care Med* 153: 1280–1284

11 The collaborative study on the genetics of asthma (CSGA) (1997) A genome-wide search for asthma susceptibility loci in ethnically diverse populations. *Nat Genetics* 15: 389–392

12 Holroyd KJ, Martinati LC, Trabetti E, Scherpbier T, Eleff SM, Boner AL, Pignatti PF, Kiser MB, Dragwa CR, Hubbard F et al (1998) Asthma and bronchial hyperresponsiveness linked to the XY long arm pseudoautosomal region. *Genomics* 52 (2): 233–235

13 Grasso L, Huang M, Sullivan CD, Messler CJ, Kiser MB, Dragwa CR, Holroyd KJ, Renauld JC, Levitt RC, Nicolaides NC (1998) Molecular analysis of human interleukin-9 receptor transcripts in peripheral blood mononuclear cells: Identification of a splice variant encoding for a nonfunctional cell surface receptor. *J Biol Chem* 273: 24016–24024

14 McLane MP, Haczku A, van de Rijn M, Weiss C, Ferrante V, MacDonald D, Renauld JC, Nicolaides NC, Holroyd KJ, Levitt RC (1998) Interleukin-9 promotes allergen-induced eosinophilic inflammation and airway hyperresponsiveness transgenic mice. *Am J Respir Cell Mol Biol* 19 (5): 713–720

15 Temann UA, Geba GP, Rankin JA, Flavell RA (1999) Expression of interleukin-9 in the lungs of transgenic mice causes airway inflammation, mast cell hyperplasia, and bronchial hyperresponsiveness. *J Exp Med* 188 (7): 1307–1320

16 Shimbara A, Christodoulopoulos P, Soussi-Gounni A, Olivenstein R, Nakamura Y, Levitt RC, Nicolaides NC, Holroyd KJ, Tsicopoulos A, Lafitte JJ et al (2000) IL-9 and its receptor in allergic and nonallergic lung disease: increased expression in asthma. *J Allergy Clin Immunol* 105: 108–115

17 Renauld J-C, Kermouni A, Vink A, Louahed J, Van Snick J (1995) Interleukin–9 and its

receptor: involvement in mast cell differentiation and T cell oncogenesis. *J Leukoc Biol* 57: 353–360

18 Louahed J, Kermouni A, Van Snick J, Renauld J-C (1995) IL-9 induces expression of granzymes and high affinity IgE receptor in murine T helper clones. *J Immunol* 154: 5061–5070

19 Eklund KK, Ghildyal N, Austen KF, Stevens RL (1993) Induction by IL-9 and suppression by IL-3 and IL-4 of the levels of chromosome 14-derived transcripts that encode late–expressed mouse mast cell proteases. *J Immunol* 151: 4266–4273

20 Dugas B, Renauld J-C, Pene J, Bonnefoy JY, Petit-Frere C, Braquet P, Bousquet J, Van Snick J, Mencia-Huerta JM (1993) Interleukin-9 potentiates the interleukin-4-induced immunoglobulin (IgG, IgM, and IgE) production by normal B lymphocytes. *Eur J Immunol* 23: 1134–1138

21 Petit-Frere C, Dugas B, Braquet P, Mencia-Huerta JM (1993) Interleukin-9 potentiates the interleukin-4 induced IgE and IgG1 release from murine B lymphocytes. *Immunology* 79: 146–151

22 Dong Q, Louahed J, Vink A, Sullivan CD, Messler CJ, Zhou Y, Haczku A, Huaux F, Arras M, Holroyd KJ et al (1999) IL-9 induces chemokine expression in lung epithelial cells and baseline airway eosinophilia in transgenic mice. *Eur J Immunol* 29 (7): 2130–2139

23 Levitt RC, McLane MP, MacDonald D, Ferrante V, Weiss C, Zhou T, Holroyd KJ, Nicolaides NC (1999) IL-9 pathway in asthma: new therapeutic targets for allergic inflammatory disorders. *J Allergy Clin Immunol* 103 (5 Pt 2): S485–S491

24 Louahed J, Toda M, Jen J, Hamid Q, Renauld J-C, Levitt RC, Nicolaides NC (2000) Interleukin-9 upregulates mucus expression in the airways. *Am J Respir Cell Mol Biol* 22: 649–656

25 McLane MP, Tepper J, Weiss C, Tomer Y, Taylor RE, Tumas D, Zhou Y, Haczku A, Nicolaides NC, Levitt RC (2000) Lung delivery of an interleukin-9 antibody treatment inhibits airway hyperresponsiveness (AHR), BAL eosinophilia, mucin production, and serum IgE elevations to natural antigens in a murine model of asthma. *J Allergy Clin Immunol* 105 (Part 2): S159 (Abstract 488 No I, presented at the AAAAI Conference)

26 Vermeesch JR, Petit P, Kermouni A, Renauld JC, Van Den Berghe H, Marynen P (1997) The IL-9 receptor gene, located in the Xq/Yq pseudoautosomal region, has an autosomal origin, escapes X inactivation and is expressed from the Y. *Hum Mol Genet* 6 (1): 1–8

Genetics of the nitric oxide synthetic pathway in asthma

Hartmut Grasemann[1] and Jeffrey M. Drazen[2]

[1]Children's Hospital, University of Essen, Hufelandstr. 55, 45122 Essen, Germany; [2]Division of Pulmonary and Critical Care Medicine, Brigham and Women's Hospital, 75 Francis Street, Boston, MA 02115, USA

Introduction

Nitric oxide (NO) is an endogenously formed biological mediator that has been shown to be involved in multiple biological processes including neurotransmission, vascular relaxation, micro-vascular permeability, host defense, and modulation of immune function [1–4]. NO is endogenously produced by a family of enzymes known as NO synthases (NOSs). Three distinct isoforms of NOS exist, each of which is encoded by a different gene localized in specific chromosomal regions in the human genome, which are 12q24.2 for neuronal NOS or NOS1 [5], 17qcen-q12 for inducible NOS or NOS2 [6], and 7q35-36 for endothelial NOS or NOS3 [7]. Each type of NOS has the capacity to catalyze the 5-electron oxidation of the semi-essential amino acid L-arginine to form L-citrulline and NO.

NOS proteins can be found in a number of different cells within the respiratory tract, including neurons, smooth muscle, and airway epithelial cells [2, 8]. The activity of NOS2, the "high-output" NOS, is transcriptionally regulated. IFNγ is most commonly associated with enhanced activation of NOS2, but other cytokines such as TNFα and IL-1β have also been shown to initiate transcription of this message, which is followed by enhanced enzyme activity in, for example, airway epithelial cells [8–10]. In contrast, transcription of NOS2 message and NOS2 enzyme activity can be decreased by corticosteroids, possibly through known NF-κB sites in the 5'-UTR of the NOS2 gene [11]. NO formation from NOS1 and NOS3, the so-called constitutively expressed NOSs, is regulated predominantly through changes in intracellular Ca^{2+} concentration. However, NOS3 messenger RNA levels can respond to mechanical stimuli such as shear stress [12, 13]; similarly, transcription of NOS1 is enhanced by multiple physical factors such as hypoxia, heat, electrical stimulation, and inflammation [14–18]. Further regulation of NOS1 activity also occurs through the variety of NOS1 transcripts that have been described. These different transcripts arise from the existence of at least nine alternative promoters, cassette exon deletions and insertions, or the use of polyadenylation signals and give rise to substantial diversity in the NOS1 message [19]. Interestingly, an interaction between NOS1 and NOS2 has been observed in rat glia cells, where tonically expressed NOS1 inhibits NOS2 expression via suppression of NF-κB [20]. In a different study with rat tissues, treatment with LPS or IFNγ induced the expression of NOS2 and decreased that of NOS1, suggesting an opposing regulatory mechanism for these two isoforms of NOS [21].

The short half-life of NO itself, in biological systems, results from rapid formation of a variety of chemical forms that can be recovered from airway lining fluid and exhaled gas [22]. Airway NO and NO metabolites have multiple, and sometimes opposing, actions that to date are not completely understood. For example, NO can be a bronchodilator through formation of nitrosothiols (SNOs) or can be converted to molecules such as peroxynitrite ($OONO^-$) with proinflammatory effects on the airways. Airway NO concentrations have been found to be elevated in patients with asthma [23–25], which is believed to be due to increased expression of NOS2 in asthma airway epithelial cells [26]. Since airway NO levels fall in response to anti-inflammatory treatment with corticosteroids or anti-leukotrienes in asthma patients [24, 25, 27], the measurement of exhaled NO has been suggested to be used as a non-invasive tool in the assessment and follow-up of airway inflammation in asthma, although the exact source of NO and the relative contribution of the three NOS isoforms to mixed airway NO in exhaled air remains unclear.

Mouse studies

To investigate the role of the distinct NOS isoforms for inflammation and airway hyperresponsiveness in asthma, studies have been performed in mice with targeted deletion of the genes encoding for these enzymes. It has been demonstrated by using a model of allergic airway inflammation that mice deficient for nos2 expressed significantly less inflammation in the airways, including infiltration of eosinophils, pulmonary edema, and plasma leakage into the airway lumen, when compared with wild-type mice [28]. In this model downregulation of NO production in the airways did not alter the type 2 cytokine-driven specific IgG1 and IgE responses, nor did it modify the production of IL-4 and IL-5 by lung T cells. There was, however, an increase in T-cell-derived IFNγ concentrations. The central role of IFNγ in this model was supported by the fact that the allergic inflammation and pathology in the nos2-deficient mice were restored after treating them during the course of sensitization against ovalbumin with antibodies against IFNγ. However, airway hyperresponsiveness to methacholine was not affected by the lack of nos2 [28]. This interesting finding was confirmed in a study with mice that had targeted deletions of one of the three nos genes, respectively, or were doubly deficient in nos1 and nos3 [29]. Although nos2 activity was significantly increased in the lungs of ovalbumin-sensi-

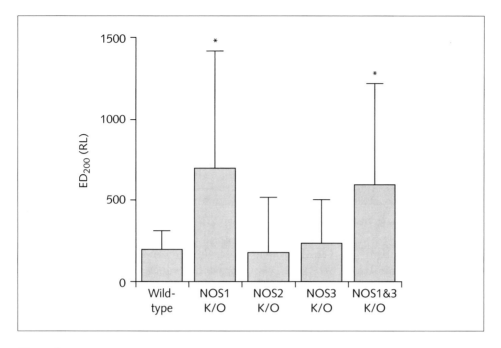

Figure 1
Airway responsiveness to methacholine measured as ED_{200} RL in anesthetized, OVA-treated wild-type mice, as well as NOS1-, NOS2-, NOS3-, and NOS1&3 knock-out (K/O) mice. Airway responsiveness was significantly reduced in NOS1- and NOS1&3-deficient mice compared with wild-type (* = p < 0.01) [29].

tized and -challenged wild-type mice and nos3-deficient mice, and nos2 activity was, as expected, undetectable in similarly treated nos2-deficient mice, airway responsiveness was not different among these groups. Remarkably, however, airway responsiveness to methacholine, in this model of allergic asthma, was significantly less in mice deficient in nos1 and those lacking nos1 and nos3 when compared with wild-type mice (Fig. 1) [29]. These results confirmed the previously reported observation of decreased airway responsiveness in naive mice with targeted deletion of the nos1 gene [30].

These findings in the mouse suggested a non-inflammatory link between the NOS1 gene and airway hyperresponsiveness, and thus we turned our attention to NOS1 as an important molecule in the pathophysiology of asthma. A number of studies in humans, which are discussed in the paragraphs below, have established a genetic link between the NOS1 locus and the diagnosis of asthma or asthma-related phenotypes.

Genome-wide scans

The gene that encodes for NOS1 in humans is localized on the long arm of chromosome 12. This region is of special interest since a number of potential candidate genes for asthma, including STAT6, IFNγ, B-cell translocation gene 1 (BTG1), stem cell factor (SCF), leukotriene A_4 hydrolase (LTA4H), insulin-like growth factor-1 (IGF1), phenylalanine hydroxylase (PAH), mast cell growth factor (MGF), the β-subunit of nuclear factor-Y (NFYβ), and the NOS1 gene, map to this chromosomal region, i.e., 12q13.12-q24.2. By using the genome-wide screening approach, multiple linkage studies have been performed in families over the past five years to identify chromosomal regions that are linked to the development of asthma. Multiple loci have been linked to asthma in these studies, but evidence of linkage to the diagnosis of asthma has been established for region 12q13-q24.2 in an Afro-Caribbean population [31], in Hispanics [32], and in distinct Caucasian populations [32–34]. This region has also been linked to total serum immunoglobulin E (IgE) in Afro-Caribbeans, in the Amish [31], and in a Caucasian population distinct from those noted above for the linkage in asthma [35]. This region has also been linked to allergic rhinitis in Afro-Caribbeans [36].

Association studies

The human NOS1 gene reveals a high degree of identity to other species in the coding region, as well as similar patterns in transcription initiation and exon usage, suggesting that it has been highly conserved throughout evolution. The NOS1 gene is one of the most complex loci known in the human genome, spanning over a region greater than 240 kb. Both NOS2 with 37 kb and NOS3 with 21 kb are significantly smaller. The 1434 amino acid human NOS1 protein is encoded by 28 exons, with the translation initiation site in exon 2 and the termination site in exon 29 [37]. Nine unique exon 1 variants exist in the 5'-flanking region that are likely utilized for transcript initiation in distinct tissues [19]. The NOS1 gene contains a number of polymorphic markers. Dinucleotide $(CA)_n$ repeat polymorphisms have been found in the 5'-flanking region of exon 1, in the 5'-portion of intron 2, and in the 5' portion of exon 29, within the 3'-UTR. A trinucleotide $(AAT)_n$ repeat is located in intron 20, and three common single-nucleotide polymorphisms (SNPs) have been detected in exons 18, 22, and 29, respectively [37, 38]. Some of these markers have been used to establish a genetic association between NOS1 and the diagnosis of asthma.

The first study to show an association between asthma and the NOS1 gene was conducted on a population with asthma and a control population identified in the United States [38]. In this study a total of 410 Caucasian asthma patients and 228 Caucasian non-asthmatic controls were screened for SNPs in exon 18, exon 22, and

Table 1 - Frequencies of allele 18 of a (CA)$_n$ repeat polymorphism in exon 29 of the NOS1 gene in asthma and control populations

	N	Allele 18	P value[a]	Odds ratio (95% CI)
Asthma	490	0.061		
Control I	350	0.119	< 0.001	0.49 (0.30–0.80)
Control II	1131	0.101	< 0.001	0.58 (0.43–0.78)

[a]*p value for asthma vs control population*

exon 29 of the NOS1 gene. Enrolled asthma patients had clinical and laboratory findings consistent with the diagnosis of asthma according to the American Thoracic Society criteria and were without significant co-morbid medical condition. The mild to moderate asthma patients in this study had a forced expiratory volume in one second (FEV$_1$) between 40% and 85% of predicted normal values after at least 8 hours without inhaled beta-agonists. They were compared with volunteers that were without asthma symptoms or atopic disease by self-report. A significant difference in allele frequency was found for the SNP in exon 29 [38]. The same group, in a different study, also reported a significant association of alleles in a (CA)$_n$ repeat polymorphism in NOS1 with the diagnosis of asthma [39]. In the CA repeat study, 490 Caucasian asthma patients that were originally recruited for a multi-center asthma medication trial conducted in the United States were compared with two different Caucasian control populations. The first controls were a cohort of 350 college students from Boston, Massachusetts, and U.S. Army recruits. The second group consisted of 1131 normal subjects from across the United States participating in the Physicians Health Study. These control individuals had reported not to have asthma in their responses to questionnaires. Allele frequencies between the two control populations were almost identical, suggesting that there was no significant population substructure difference. Significant differences in allele frequencies, however, were found between asthmatics and controls. The (CA)$_{18}$ allele was significantly less common in asthmatics (0.06 vs 0.12, $p < 0.001$). This allele, with an odds ratio of 0.49 (95% CI 0.34–0.69), thus seems to be protective from asthma (Tab. 1). Although the genome-wide studies in Caucasians had found evidence for linkage of both asthma and IgE levels to chromosomal region 12q14-q24, no association with serum IgE was found in the case-control association study, suggesting that a second gene in that region accounts for high total serum IgE levels [39]. The findings of an IgE-independent association of NOS1 with asthma was recently confirmed in a study with 300 individuals from Britain using a genetic marker in intron 2 of NOS1 [40]. The difference in allele frequency was in the range of the American association

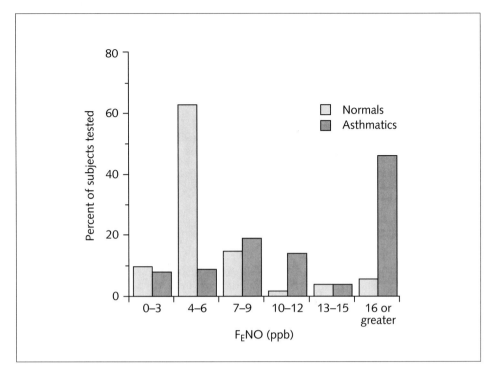

Figure 2
Distribution of mixed expired NO (FeNO) in parts per billion (ppb) in a cohort of patients with asthma and controls [25].

study with an odds ratio of 2.08 (95% CI 1.20–3.57). Interestingly, the British population was also screened for a polymorphism in the NOS2 and NOS3 gene, respectively, but no association between these genes and asthma could be found [40].

Airway nitric oxide

Elevated concentrations of NO in exhaled air (F_ENO) are now well-established phenotypic markers of asthma. In the absence of asthma-provoking events or asthma treatment, F_ENO remains relatively fixed over time in individual patients. However, when looking at the distribution of individual values, F_ENO is highly variable and there is considerable overlap between asthmatics and normals, with a fraction of asthmatics having low levels of F_ENO that are characteristic of normal subjects (Fig. 2) [23–25]. Although the molecular source of the NO in exhaled air remains unknown, data from mouse models indicate that nos1 contributes substantially to

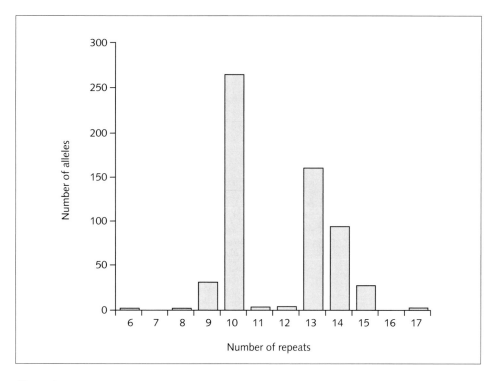

Figure 3
Allelic distribution of an AAT repeat polymorphism in intron 20 of the NOS1 gene in 305 non-asthmatic control individuals [41].

F_ENO [30]. Given the well-established association between the size of trinucleotide repeats and several human neuro-muscular conditions, a study was performed to investigate the relation of various alleles at a trinucleotide repeat polymorphism in the NOS1 gene and F_ENO in asthma [41]. In this study 97 patients with mild asthma were genotyped for an $(AAT)_n$ repeat polymorphism in intron 20 of NOS1. Measurement of F_ENO in these patients was performed in accordance with ATS guidelines. At the time of study the patients had used neither inhaled nor systemic corticosteroids within the preceding 30 days. Among these individuals nine distinct alleles ranging from 8 to 17 AAT repeats were identified. Interestingly, the relative frequency of the various alleles was bimodally distributed, with allele 10 at the lower portion and alleles 13 and 14 at the higher portion of the distribution, being the predominant alleles at this locus (Fig. 3). When segregating the patients into two groups, one consisting of individuals harboring at least one allele with fewer than 12 repeats, and the other consisting of individuals harboring two alleles with at least 12 repeats, significant differences in F_ENO were found. Both mean F_ENO

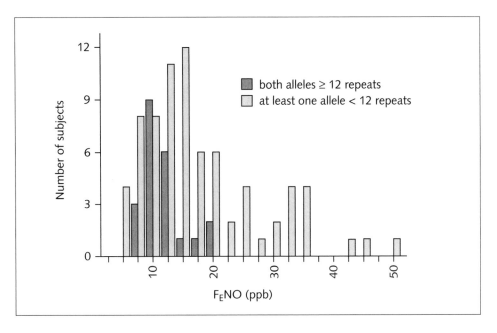

Figure 4

Distribution of expired NO (F_ENO) in 97 asthmatic individuals divided into two subgroups based on allele size of an intronic AAT-repeat polymorphism in the NOS1 gene [41].

($p < 0.0001$) and variability around the mean ($p < 0.00001$) were significantly lower in individuals with a high number of repeats (Fig. 4). Since low F_ENO is a characteristic of non-asthmatic normal individuals, the authors then genotyped 305 Caucasian controls and 495 Caucasian asthmatics and found the same alleles associated with low F_ENO in asthmatics to be significantly more common in healthy individuals than in asthmatics ($p < 0.01$) [41]. These data are consistent with the considerable evidence that neural mechanisms in general and NO in particular contribute to the pathophysiology and symptomatology of asthma. It is conceivable that patients with two high AAT repeat number alleles in NOS1 have dysfunction of nitridergic nerves and that this dysfunction accounts for their lower and less-variant mean F_ENO. An effect of intronic trinucleotide repeat size on neural bronchomotor control may be explained by the observation that trinucleotide repeats play an important role in the pathogenesis of neurodegenerative diseases, such as myotonic dystrophy, Huntington's disease, spinocerebellar ataxia, and fragile X syndrome [42, 43]. For example, in spinocerebellar ataxia, a difference of only one trinucleotide repeat in intronic DNA makes the difference between neural dysfunction and its absence in the context of total repeat numbers in the order of 20 [44].

The complex interaction of inflammation and neural control of airways, with inflammatory mediators affecting neurotransmittion and neurotransmitters in turn modulating the inflammatory response in the airways, is well known. In addition to the classic cholinergic and adrenergic neural systems, nonadrenergic noncholinergic (NANC) pathways, in which NO has been recognized to be the main neurotransmitter, are present in the airways and modulate bronchomotor tone, for example, in the induced bronchodilatatory response [45]. Thus, one component of the neurogenic regulation of asthma may be NOS1-derived NO, which, along with the NO derived from other NO synthases, may be variably involved in airway inflammation. Genetic variants in other genes contributing to this complex interaction, that have either not been found yet or have not been studied *in extensio*, such as a bi-allelic variant within the NOS2 gene promotor, may have an important impact on this neuro-inflammatory interaction in asthma.

References

1   Moncada S, Higgs A (1993) The L-arginine-nitric oxide pathway. *N Engl J Med* 329: 2002–2012

2   Barnes PJ, Belvisi MG (1993) Nitric oxide and lung disease. *Thorax* 48: 1034–1043

3   Michel T, Feron O (1997) Nitric oxide synthases: which, where, how, and why? *J Clin Invest* 100: 2146–2152

4   Nathan C (1997) Inducible nitric oxide synthase: what difference does it make? *J Clin Invest* 100: 2417–2423

5   Xu W, Gorman P, Sheer D, Bates G, Kishimoto J, Lizhi L, Emson P (1993) Regional localization of the gene coding for human brain nitric oxide synthase (NOS1) to chromosome 12q24.2-24.31by fluorescent *in situ* hybridization. *Cytogenet Cell Genet* 64: 62–63

6   Chartrain NA, Geller DA, Koty PP, Sitrin NF, Nussler AK, Hoffmann EP, Billiar TR, Hutchinson NI, Mudgett JS (1994) Molecular cloning, structure, and chromosomal localization of the human inducible nitric oxide synthase gene. *J Biol Chem* 269: 6765–6772

7   Marsden PA, Heng HHQ, Scherer SW, Stewart RJ, Hall AV, Shi XM, Tsui LC, Schappert KT (1993) Structure and chromosomal localization of the human constitutive endothelial nitric oxide synthase gene. *J Biol Chem* 268: 17478–17488

8   Asano K, Chee CB, Gaston B, Lilly CM, Gerard G, Drazen JM, Stamler JS (1994) Constitutive and inducible nitric oxide synthase gene expression, regulation, and activity in human lung epithelial cells. *Proc Natl Acad Sci USA* 91: 10089–10093

9   Robbins RA, Barnes PJ, Springall DR, Warren JB, Kwon OJ, Buttery LD, Wilson AJ, Geller DA, Polak JM (1994) Expression of inducible nitric oxide in human lung epithelial cells. *Biochem Biophys Res Commun* 203: 209–218

10 Gutierrez HH, Pitt BR, Schwarz M, Watkins SC, Lowenstein C, Caniggia I, Chumley P,

Freeman BA (1995) Pulmonary alveolar epithelial inducible NO synthase gene expression: regulation by inflammatory mediators. *Am J Physiol* 268: L501–508

11 Xie QW, Kashiwabara Y, Nathan C (1994) Role of transcription factor NF-kappa B/Rel in induction of nitric oxide synthase. *J Biol Chem* 269: 4705–4708

12 Nishida K, Harrison DG, Navas JP, Fisher AA, Dockery SP, Uematsu M, Nerem RM, Alexander RW, Murphy TJ (1992) Molecular cloning and characterization of the constitutive bovine aortic endothelial cell nitric oxide synthase. *J Clin Invest* 90: 2092–2096

13 Awolesi MA, Widmann MD, Sessa WC, Sumpio BE (1994) Cyclic strain increases endothelial nitric oxide synthase activity. *Surgery* 116: 439–444

14 Sharma HS, Westman J, Alm P, Sjoquist PO, Cervos-Navarro, Nyberg F (1997) Involvement of nitric oxide in the pathophysiology of acute heat stress in the rat. Influence of a new antioxidant compound H-290/51. *Ann NY Acad Sci* 813: 581–590

15 Reiser PJ, Kline WO, Vaghy PL (1997) Induction of neuronal type nitric oxide synthase in skeletal muscle by chronic electrical stimulation *in vivo*. *J Appl Physiol* 82: 1250–1255

16 Shaul PW, North AJ, Brannon TS, Ujiie K, Wells LB, Nisen PA, Lowenstein CJ, Snyder SH, Star RA (1995) Prolonged *in vivo* hypoxia enhances nitric oxide synthase type I and type III gene expression in adult rat lung. *Am J Respir Cell Mol Biol* 13: 167–174

17 Prabhakar NR, Rao S, Premkumar D, Pieramici SF, Kumar GK, Kalaria RK (1996) Regulation of neuronal nitric oxide synthase gene expression by hypoxia. Role of nitric oxide in respiratory adaptation to low pO_2. *Adv Exp Med Biol* 410: 345–348

18 Calza L, Giardino L, Pozza M, Micera A, Aloe L (1997) Time-course changes of nerve growth factor, corticotropin-releasing hormone, and nitric oxide synthase isoforms and their possible role in the development of inflammatory response in experimental allergic encephalomyelitis. *Proc Natl Acad Sci USA* 94: 3368–3373

19 Wang Y, Newton DC, Robb GB, Kau CL, Miller TL, Cheung AH, Hall AV, VanDamme S, Wilcox JN, Marsden PA (1999) RNA diversity has profound effects on the translation of neuronal nitric oxide synthase. *Proc Natl Acad Sci USA* 96: 12150–12155

20 Togashi H, Sasaki M, Frohman E, Taira E, Ratan RR, Dawson TM, Dawson VL (1997) Neuronal (type I) nitric oxide synthase regulates nuclear factor kappaB activity and immunologic (type II) nitric oxide synthase expression. *Proc Natl Acad Sci USA* 94: 2676–2680

21 Bandyopadhyay A, Chakder S, Rattan S (1997) Regulation of inducible and neuronal nitric oxide synthase gene expression by interferon-gamma and VIP. *Am J Physiol* 272: C1790–1797

22 Gaston B, Drazen JM, Loscalzo J, Stamler JS (1994) The biology of nitrogen oxides in the airways. *Am J Respir Crit Care Med* 149: 538–551

23 Persson MG, Zetterstrom O, Agrenius V, Ihre E, Gustafsson LE (1994) Single-breath nitric oxide measurements in asthmatic patients and smokers. *Lancet* 343: 146–147

24 Kharitonov SA, Yates D, Robbins RA, Logan-Sinclair R, Shinebourne EA, Barnes PJ (1994) Increased nitric oxide in exhaled air of asthmatic patients. *Lancet* 343: 133–135

25 Massaro AF, Gaston B, Kita D, Fanta C, Stamler JS, Drazen JM (1995) Expired nitric

oxide levels during treatment of acute asthma. *Am J Respir Crit Care Med* 152: 800–803

26   Hamid Q, Springall DR, Riveros-Moreno V, Chanez P, Howarth P, Redington A, Bousquet J, Godard P, Holgate S, Polak JM (1993) Induction of nitric oxide synthase in asthma. *Lancet* 342: 1510–1513

27   Bisgaard H, Loland L, Oj JA (1999) NO in exhaled air of asthmatic children is reduced by the leukotriene receptor antagonist montelukast. *Am J Respir Crit Care Med* 160: 1227–1231

28   Xiong Y, Karupiah G, Hogan SP, Foster PS, Ramsay AJ (1999) Inhibition of allergic airway inflammation in mice lacking nitric oxide synthase 2. *J Immunol* 162: 445–452

29   De Sanctis GT, MacLean JA, Hamada K, Mehta S, Scott J, Jiao A, Yandava CN, Kobzic L, Wolyniec WW, Fabian A et al (1999) Contribution of nitric oxide synthases 1, 2, and 3 to airway hyperresponsiveness and inflammation in a murine model of asthma. *J Exp Med* 189: 1621–1630

30   De Sanctis GT, Mehta S, Kobzik L, Yandava C, Jiao A, Huang PL, Drazen JM (1997) Contribution of type I NOS to expired gas NO and bronchial responsiveness in mice. *Am J Physiol* 273: L883–L888

31   Barnes KC, Neely JD, Duffy DL, Freidhoff LR, Breazeale DR, Schou C, Naidu RP, Levett PN, Renault B, Kucherlapati R et al (1996) Linkage of asthma and serum IgE concentration to markers on chromosome 12q: evidence from Afro-Caribbean and Caucasian populations. *Genomics* 37: 41–50

32   The Collaborative Study on the Genetics of Asthma (CSGA) (1997) A genome-wide search for asthma susceptibility loci in ethnically diverse populations. *Nat Genet* 15: 389–392

33   Thomas NS, Wilkinson J, Holgate ST (1997) The candidate gene approach to the genetics of asthma and allergy. *Am J Respir Crit Care Med* 156: S144–S151

34   Ober C, Cox NJ, Abney M, Di Rienzo A, Lander ES, Changyaleket B, Gidley H, Kurtz B, Lee J, Nance M et al and The Collaborative Study on the Genetics of Asthma (1998) Genome-wide search for asthma susceptibility loci in a founder population. *Hum Mol Genet* 7: 1393–1398

35   Nickel R, Wahn U, Hizawa N, Maestri N, Duffy DL, Barnes KC, Beyer K, Forster J, Bergmann R, Zepp F et al (1997) Evidence for linkage of chromosome 12q15-q24.1 markers to high total serum IgE concentrations in children of the German multicenter allergy study. *Genomics* 46: 159–162

36   Barnes KC, Freidhoff LR, Nickel R, Chiu YF, Juo SH, Hizawa N, Naidu RP, Ehrlich E, Duffy DL, Schou C et al (1999) Dense mapping of chromosome 12q13.12-q23.3 and linkage to asthma and allergy. *J Allergy Clin Immunol* 104: 485–491

37   Hall AV, Antoniou H, Wang Y, Cheung AH, Arbus AM, Olson SL, Lu WC, Kau CL, Marsden PA (1994) Structural organization of the human neuronal nitric oxide synthase gene (NOS1). *J Biol Chem* 269: 33082–33090

38   Grasemann H, Yandava CN, Drazen JM (1999) Neuronal NO synthase (NOS1) is a major candidate gene for asthma. *Clin Exp Allergy* 29 (Suppl 4): 39–41

39 Grasemann H, Yandava CN, Storm van's Gravesande K, Deykin A, Pillari A, Ma J, Sonna LA, Lilly C, Stampfer MJ, Israel E et al (2000) A neuronal NO synthase (NOS1) gene polymorphism is associated with asthma. *Biochem Biophys Res Commun* 272: 391–394

40 Gao PS, Kawada H, Kasamatsu T, Mao XQ, Roberts MH, Miyamoto Y, Yoshimura M, Saitoh Y, Yasue H, Nakao K et al (2000) Variants of NOS1, NOS2, and NOS3 genes in asthmatics. *Biochem Biophys Res Commun* 267: 361–363

41 Wechsler ME, Grasemann H, Deykin A, Silverman EK, Yandava CN, Israel E, Wand M, Drazen JM (2000) Exhaled nitric oxide in patients with asthma: association with NOS1 genotype. *Am J Respir Crit Care Med* 162: 2172–2176

42 Timchenko LT, Caskey CT (1996) Trinucleotide repeat disorders in humans: discussions of mechanisms and medical issues. *FASEB J* 10: 1589–1597

43 Martin JB (1999) Molecular pathobiology of neurodegenerative diseases. *N Engl J Med* 340: 1970–1980

44 Pearson CE, Sinden RR (1998) Trinucleotide repeat DNA structures: dynamic mutations from dynamic DNA. *Curr Opin Struct Biol* 8: 321–330

45 Belvisi MG, Ward JK, Mitchell JA, Barnes PJ (1995) Nitric oxide as a neurotransmitter in human airways. *Arch Int Pharmacodyn* 329: 97–110

Genetic regulation of leukotriene production and activity

I. Sayers[1] and A. P. Sampson[2]

[1]Human Genetics and [2]Respiratory Cell & Molecular Biology Research Division, Southampton General Hospital, Tremona Road, Southampton, SO16 6YD, UK

Introduction

Leukotrienes (LTs) have been identified as critical mediators of airway narrowing and eosinophilia in bronchial asthma. They potently contract human bronchial smooth muscle, promote mucus secretion and impair muciliary clearance, increase vascular permeability leading to airway oedema, and, specifically, chemoattract human eosinophils *in vitro* and *in vivo*. In view of the importance of these lipid mediators in the pathogenesis of asthma, substantial effort has been directed at elucidating the mechanisms that regulate their production by the 5-lipoxygenase pathway and those that mediate their effects [1]. This work led directly to the development of a series of LT modifier drugs that show clinical efficiency in asthma and represent the first new form of asthma treatment in 25 years [2, 3].

This chapter will review the current understanding of the genetic mechanisms that regulate leukotriene production and activity, including an appraisal of the pharmacogenetics of the recently introduced LT modifier drugs. Post-transcriptional and post-translational mechanisms involved in LT production and/or activity will not be addressed in this review.

The 5-lipoxygenase pathway

Following cell activation by allergen or alternative stimuli, intracellular calcium levels increase, initiating a series of membrane events leading to the activation of phospholipase A_2 (PLA_2). PLA_2 liberates arachidonic acid (AA), the initial substrate of the 5-LO pathway, by catalysing the hydrolysis of nuclear envelope phospholipids. AA is a substrate for the cyclooxygenase pathway that generates thromboxane and prostaglandins and for the 5-LO pathway that generates LTs. Free arachidonate binds to 5-lipoxygenase activating protein (FLAP), an integral perinuclear membrane protein, and is presented to 5-lipoxygenase (5-LO) (Fig. 1) [4].

The Hereditary Basis of Allergic Diseases, edited by Stephen T. Holgate and John W. Holloway
© 2002 Birkhäuser Verlag Basel/Switzerland

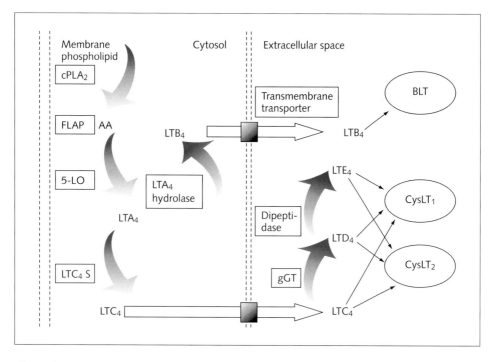

Figure 1

Principal enzymes of the 5-lipoxygenase pathway.

cPLA$_2$, cytosolic PLA$_2$; 5-LO, 5-lipoxygenase; FLAP, 5-lipoxygenase activating protein; AA, arachidonic acid; LTC$_4$ S, LTC$_4$ synthase; gGT, γ-glutamyl-transpeptidase; BLT, LTB$_4$ receptor; CysLT$_1$, CysLT$_2$, cysteinyl leukotriene receptor subtypes (see text).

AA is metabolised by 5-LO to form the unstable epoxide intermediate LTA$_4$ *via* a two-step process involving the initial oxygenation of AA to form 5-hydroperoxy-6,8,11,14-eicosatetraenoic acid (5-HPETE) followed by conversion to LTA$_4$ [4]. Depending on the presence of the appropriate enzymes, LTA$_4$ can be conjugated with reduced glutathione by LTC$_4$ synthase to produce LTC$_4$, the first cysteinyl-leukotriene (cys-LT) family member generated in the pathway. Alternatively, LTA$_4$ can be converted to LTB$_4$ under the action of LTA$_4$ hydrolase. These actions are cell-type dependent, with eosinophils and mast cells favouring LTC$_4$ production and neutrophils and macrophages favouring LTB$_4$ production. LTB$_4$ is a dihydroxy acid with potent neutrophil chemoattractant properties, and both LTB$_4$ and LTC$_4$ are secreted from the cell *via* a carrier-mediated process. LTC$_4$ is further metabolised to produce the other cys-LT family members, LTD$_4$ and LTE$_4$, by the action of γ-glutamyl transpeptidase and dipeptidase, respectively (Fig. 1).

5-LO and FLAP are thought to be restricted mainly to cells of myeloid lineage, including neutrophils, eosinophils, monocytes-macrophages, and mast cells, so *de novo* production of LTA_4 is limited to these cells [5–7]. The terminal enzymes LTA_4 hydrolase and LTC_4 synthase are more widely distributed; therefore, transcellular synthesis may occur in which neutrophils and other cells that express 5-LO/FLAP donate LTA_4 to other cells such as platelets and endothelial cells that express the terminal enzymes, leading to additional production of LTB_4 and cysLTs *via* cell-cell interaction.

LTs produce their effects *via* interaction with specific membrane receptors on target cells. The receptors for cys-LTs (LTC_4, LTD_4, LTE_4) and LTB_4 are distinct; the LTB_4 receptor is designated BLT, and two sub-types of cys-LT receptor have been designated, $CysLT_1$ and $CysLT_2$.

Effects of leukotrienes on airway function

Leukotrienes elicit a number of effects that mimic the pathophysiology of airway inflammation, including bronchial smooth muscle contraction, increased mucus secretion, vasodilation, increased microvascular permeability, and eosinophil recruitment. The cys-LTs are potent bronchoconstrictors, with LTC_4 and LTD_4 being approximately 1000-fold more potent than histamine on a molar basis in both normal and asthmatic volunteers [8–10]. The response is slower in onset and longer-lived than that of histamine, which led to the original designation of variable mixtures of cys-LTs as "slow-reacting substance of anaphylaxis" (SRS-A).

The cys-LTs stimulate mucus secretion and increase vascular permeability in human airways [11], which combine with bronchial smooth muscle contraction to cause airway occlusion in severe disease. In normals and asthmatics, cys-LTs increase non-specific bronchial responsiveness (BHR), an important marker of the asthma phenotype. Inhaled LTE_4 elicits bronchospasm in asthmatics at doses nearly 200-fold lower than in normal subjects, illustrating the uniquely heightened responsiveness of subjects with asthma to this cys-LT [12].

In asthma, the numbers of eosinophils in the circulation and in bronchoalveolar lavage (BAL) fluid correlate with disease severity [13]. Eosinophils are a significant source of LTC_4 and a wide variety of cytokines and granule-associated proteins that modulate the inflammatory response in the airways. LTC_4, LTD_4, and LTE_4 have selective chemoattractant activity for eosinophils both *in vitro* and *in vivo* [14, 15]. Although LT measurements in blood are not well established, plasma levels of LTC_4 and LTD_4 in blood have been reported to increase during episodes of wheezing [16], and LTC_4 levels in BAL fluid clearly increase following inhaled allergen challenge in atopic asthmatics [17]. Similarly, elevated levels of urinary LTE_4 have been observed in atopic asthmatics following allergen challenge, in aspirin-intolerant asthmatics (AIA), and in spontaneous severe asthma exacerbations [18, 19]. In AIA patients,

elevated LTC_4 levels in the nasal lavage have been observed following aspirin inges-
tion compared with controls and aspirin-tolerant asthmatics (ATA) [20, 21]. A dose-
response relationship between cys-LT levels in nasal lavage fluid and rhinitic symptoms has been observed in ragweed-sensitive allergic rhinitis patients following
increasing doses of ragweed [22]. These findings provide evidence for the role of
cys-LTs in the pathogenesis of asthma.

Although less clearly implicated in asthma, LTB_4 has been implicated in inflammatory processes, including potent neutrophil chemotaxis, the promotion of neu-
trophil-endothelial adhesion [23], and as a stimulator of cytokine production by T
cells (interleukin-5 (IL-5)) [24] and monocytes (IL-6) [25]. LTB_4 binds to cell-sur-
face BLT receptors, and may also bind to the transcription factor PPARα resulting
in gene activation [26]. More recently LTB_4 has been shown to mediate the induction of NF-κB and IL-8 by histamine in human bronchial epithelial cells [27].

The role of LTs is thought to be more pronounced in a subgroup of asthmatic
patients with aspirin-intolerant asthma (AIA), also known as aspirin-sensitive asthma (ASA). In these patients, inhibition of cyclooxygenase by aspirin and other
NSAIDs triggers a surge of cys-LT production, probably by removing PGE_2-depen-
dent inhibition, leading to acute bronchosconstriction, often accompanied by
rhinoconjunctival and dermal symptoms. AIA patients also have chronically elevated cys-LT production, as detected by urinary LTE_4, associated with generally severe
steroid-dependent, chronic asthma. A persistent five-fold elevation in the number of
cells expressing the terminal enzyme for cys-LT production, LTC_4 synthase, has been
demonstrated in AIA lung biopsies compared with ATA and normal subjects; the
increase was due partly to increased eosinophils and partly to an increased proportion of eosinophils expressing the enzyme. The increased LTC_4 synthase expression
correlated significantly with elevated cys-LT levels in BAL fluid and with bronchial
hyperresponsiveness to inhaled lysine aspirin [28].

In conclusion, the evidence is now overwhelming that cys-LT plays a critical role
in asthma, including defined roles in bronchoconstriction and eosinophilia [29]. The
clinical efficiency in asthma of drugs that modify LT activity has reinforced this central role.

Leukotriene receptors

LTB_4 and the cys-LTs exert their activities by interacting with cellular receptors.
LTB_4 acts at a G-protein coupled receptor (GPCR) termed BLT, resulting in proinflammatory actions including neutrophil chemotaxis [30, 31]. The BLT receptor has
been identified on multiple cell types including human leukocytes, spleen, and thymus [31]. Differential binding sites have been identified for the BLT receptor with
nanomolar and sub-nanomolar affinities [32]; the high-affinity site mediates the
potent neutrophil chemotaxis associated with LTB_4, and the low-affinity site is

implicated in neutrophil activation. BLT activation is associated with increases in intracellular calcium and inhibition of adenylate cyclase. Intriguingly, BLT has been identified as a co-receptor for HIV infection, suggesting multiple roles for this GPCR [33]. The gene that encodes BLT has been cloned and sequenced and is described in detail below.

At least two cys-LT receptors (CysLT$_1$ and CysLT$_2$) have been identified pharmacologically [34]. Most of the biological functions of cys-LTs, including bronchoconstriction, are mediated *via* the CysLT$_1$ receptor, while CysLT$_2$ may mediate some vascular actions. The CysLT$_1$ receptor is the target for several leukotriene receptor antagonist drugs including montelukast (Singulair) and zafirlukast (Accolate), which have shown clinical efficiency in asthma, as described below. Prior to cloning of the cys-LT receptors, isolated guinea pig lung membranes and cell lines, including the human monocytic cell line U-937, which has a high number of LTD$_4$ binding sites, were used to characterise these receptors. Potencies of LTD$_4$ > LTC$_4$ > LTE$_4$ >> LXA$_4$ were observed for CysLT$_1$ [30], and it was shown that receptor activation resulted in calcium elevation. The second cys-LT receptor (CysLT$_2$) was identified on guinea pig trachea, sheep bronchus, and human pulmonary and saphenous vein preparations, with potencies LTC$_4$ = LTD$_4$ >> LTE$_4$.

The cloning of CysLT$_1$ [35, 36] and CysLT$_2$ [37] confirmed many of the observations using isolated tissue and has now paved the way for the identification of genetic mechanisms involved in the regulation of cys-LT receptor function.

Leukotriene modifier drugs

Three forms of anti-asthma drugs have been developed that target the 5-LO pathway: (1) 5-LO inhibitors; (2) FLAP inhibitors, together described as LT synthesis inhibitors (LTSI); and (3) CysLT$_1$ receptor antagonists, known as LTRA. The 5-LO inhibitor zileuton is available in the US; elsewhere, LTRAs including montelukast (Singulair), pranlukast (Onon), and zafirlukast (Accolate) are used in clinical medicine and have shown great potential across the whole spectrum of asthma severity [2, 38]. Bronchoprovocation studies have shown that LTSI or LTRA partly or wholly block constrictor responses to a wide range of asthma triggers, including inhaled allergen, platelet activating factor (PAF), exercise, cold air, sulphur dioxide (SO$_2$), adenosine 5'-monophosphate (AMP), and nonsteroidal anti-inflammatory drugs (NSAIDs) [39]. In addition, 10–15% improvements in baseline lung function, with 25–60% improvements in secondary outcome measures, including symptom scores, nighttime awakenings, use of rescue medication (β-agonists and glucocorticoids), and days absent from work or school, have been reported in multiple-dose trials in allergic and non-allergic asthma [40]. Selective BLT antagonists have also been developed, such as LY 293111, which significantly blocks neutrophil influx following inhaled allergen challenge but has no effect on lung function or bronchial responsiveness, questioning the role of LTB_4/BLT in asthma [41].

The clinical effectiveness of anti-leukotriene drugs has highlighted the central role of leukotrienes in asthma pathogenesis, but it is not clear why some patients respond extremely well while others show no significant clinical improvement. This heterogeneity in drug response may have a genetic component. The remainder of this chapter will review current understanding of the immunogenetic regulation of LT production and activity including the pharmacogenetics of LT modifier drugs.

Immunopharmacological regulation of LT production

Over-production of cys-LT in asthma depends on a number of factors, including the variable capacity of individual leukocytes to generate cys-LT when stimulated and the numbers of each leukocyte sub-type present in the airway wall. Bronchial biopsy studies show that elevated expression of 5-LO pathway enzymes in the airway wall in symptomatic asthmatics is particularly associated with increased eosinophils and monocytes [28, 42].

Blood eosinophils from asthmatic patients synthesize 5- to 10-fold greater amounts of cys-LTs than those from normal subjects [43–45], and this can be mimicked *in vitro* by treatment of normal eosinophils with eosinophilopoietic cytokines including IL-3, IL-5, and GM-CSF [46–49]. In CD34+ umbilical cord blood cells forced to differentiate into eosinophils by culture with IL-5 and IL-3, the capacity to synthesise cys-LT is acquired following sequential expression of $cPLA_2$, 5-LO, FLAP, and LTC_4 synthase over 14 to 28 days [50]. In human blood leukocytes, *in vitro* priming of LT synthesis by IL-3, IL-5, and GM-CSF may involve $cPLA_2$ activation that leads to enhanced arachidonate availability [51, 52] followed by gene transcription and protein synthesis of 5-LO and/or FLAP [53–61]. *In vivo*, upregulation of 5-LO and FLAP expression accounts for the marked increase in LTB_4 synthesis observed as blood monocytes differentiate into alveolar macrophages [62], and excess FLAP expression is observed in blood eosinophils of mild asthmatic subjects [61].

In eosinophils, the cytokine with the most specific effect on promoting terminal differentiation and on enhancing survival, migration, degranulation, and cys-LT synthesis is IL-5 [49]. IL-5 is synthesized by T cells and mast cells in the asthmatic airway [63], and is detectable in the plasma of symptomatic asthmatics [64, 65]. IL-5 acts on eosinophils *via* a receptor composed of a specific α unit (60–80 kDa), and a 120 kDa β unit that is common to IL-3 and GM-CSF receptors [65a]. Binding of IL-5 to its receptor causes activation of cytosolic tyrosine kinases, including the Janus kinase JAK2, which activates the nuclear transcription factor Stat1, and tyrosine kinase activity is essential for priming of eosinophil effector function by IL-5 [66, 67].

In resting human leukocytes, 5-LO is largely cytosolic in distribution, but in cells that have undergone tissue recruitment and differentiation, a significant proportion of cellular 5-LO localises to the nuclear euchromatin [68, 69]. 5-LO translocation is associated with enhanced LT synthesis in cytokine-primed, adherent, and tissue-differentiated eosinophils, neutrophils, and macrophages [61, 68, 69] but with a reduction in cys-LT synthesis in eosinophils adhered to fibronectin for 2 h [70]. Although IL-5 priming is not Ca^{2+}-dependent, low concentrations of calcium ionophore mimic IL-5 priming. In leukocytes activated by high concentrations of ionophore, a rapid translocation of 5-LO to the nuclear envelope occurs that also depends on tyrosine kinase activity and on a functional microtubule system and is associated with accumulation of phosphorylated 5-LO [71–73].

The effects of glucocorticoids on the 5-LO pathway are complex. *In vitro*, glucocorticoids may suppress eicosanoid synthesis in alveolar macrophages by inducing the expression of lipocortin-1, an inhibitor of $cPLA_2$ [74], but their effects in blood leukocytes are highly-dependent on cell type and activation status. Anti-inflammatory glucocorticoid therapy reduces IL-5 expression *in vivo* and suppresses airway eosinophilia in asthma [64, 75]. Paradoxically, glucocorticoids enhance FLAP expression in human eosinophils, neutrophils, monocytes, and monocytic THP-1 cells *in vitro* [61, 76, 77]. In human blood monocytes and monocytic THP-1 cells, but not in eosinophils or neutrophils, this is accompanied by increased ionophore-stimulated LT synthesis. The effects of dexamethasone on FLAP expression may therefore be counter-balanced by inhibition of the activity and/or expression of proximal and distal enzymes in the 5-LO pathway, particularly $cPLA_2$ [74]. The activity of the terminal enzyme in the cys-LT pathway, LTC_4 synthase, is not altered by IL-5 or GM-CSF in an eosinophilic substrain of HL-60 cells [78]. Overall, the inconsistent effect of dexamethasone on cys-LT synthesis in leukocytes *in vitro* is consistent with the failure of systemic glucocorticoid therapy to inhibit *in vivo* leukotriene synthesis in normal and asthmatic patients [79, 80].

Genetic regulation of LT production and activity

Asthma is a complex, multifactorial genetic disorder, but genes that regulate LT production and activity provide excellent candidates for asthma susceptibility and severity [81]. Multiple gene products have a potential role in the modulation of LT production, including the genes encoding enzymes, transcription factors, transport proteins, and receptors. This chapter will concentrate on the primary candidates including genes encoding for the enzymes of the 5-LO pathway and for LT receptors including BLT, $CysLT_1$ and $CysLT_2$ (Tab. 1). In addition to genetic factors, the microenvironment can have profound influences on LT production, and therefore genetic predisposition in combination with a specific microenvironment (cytokines, growth factors, etc.) is likely to regulate LT production and activity (Fig. 2).

Table 1 - Candidate genes involved in the regulation of leukotriene production and activity

Gene	Name	Chromosome location	Linkage to asthma/atopy	Poly- morphism	Refs.
PLA2G4	Phospholipase A_2 (cPLA$_2$ type IV)	1q25	Yes	(CA) and (A) repeats	[87]
PLA2G2A	Phospholipase A_2 (sPLA$_2$ type IIA)	1p35	Yes	?	
ALOX5	Arachidonate-5- lipoxygenase (5-LO)	10	Yes	Sp-1/Egr-1 Binding sites −1706 G/A −1761 G/A	[98]
ALOX5AP	Arachidonate-5-lipoxygenase activating protein (FLAP)	13q12.3	Yes	?	
LTC4S	LTC$_4$ synthase	5q35	Yes	−444 A/C AP2 site	[117]
LTA4H	LTA$_4$ hydrolase	12q22	Yes	Exon 1 102 G/T 114 C/T	[108]
BLT	LTB$_4$ receptor	14q11.2-12	Yes	?	
CysLT1R	CysLT$_1$ receptor	Xq13-21	No	Leu206Ser Gly300Ser Phe309Phe	[137]
CysLT2R	CysLT$_2$ receptor	13q14	Yes	?	

Candidate genes are listed with chromosomal locations and previously identified polymorphisms. Chromosomal regions linked to asthma and atopy phenotypes in genome-wide scans are highlighted [81].

Molecular biology of the 5-LO pathway

Phospholipase A_2 (PLA$_2$)

The substrate for LT synthesis, arachidonic acid, is generated from membrane phospholipids by PLA$_2$. It is unclear whether isozymes of cytosolic (85 kDa) or secretory (14 kDa) PLA$_2$ are more important in LT synthesis in human lung mast cells and eosinophils. In monocytes, cPLA$_2$ is not required for LT synthesis, but in alveolar macrophages, both cPLA$_2$ and sPLA$_2$ are involved, with cPLA$_2$ playing a greater role in asthmatic patients than in normal subjects [82]. Human eosinophils, which are the predominant source of cys-LTs in the lungs of persistent asthmatics [28], express very large amounts of sPLA$_2$. cPLA$_2$ has been implicated directly in the

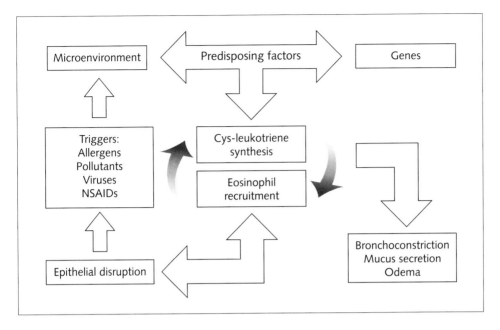

Figure 2
Leukotriene synthesis and activity is determined by gene-microenvironment interactions (adapted from [120]).

allergic response using cPLA$_2$-deficient mice that displayed a decreased production of eicosanoids and platelet-activating factor and a significant reduction in anaphylactic responses and bronchial reactivity to methacholine [83]. This evidence, and the findings that cPLA$_2$ functions in the cytosol rather than the extracellular space and that it selectively cleaves arachidonic acid from membrane vesicles and translocates from cytosolic fractions to membrane vesticular in the presence of calcium [84], the site of FLAP and LTC$_4$ synthase activity, provides evidence that this form is most likely to have a role on leukotriene production.

The cytosolic PLA$_2$ gene (PLA2G4) is located at chromosome 1q25 [85], and the cDNA has been isolated, encoding for a protein of 749 amino acids [86]. The genomic structure of cPLA$_2$ is not known, but the 5' UTR of the gene has been investigated. The 5' flanking region of the PLA2G4 gene has been characterised, and transcription factor binding sites have been identified, including NF-κB, NF-IL-6, AP-1, PEA3, interferon-γ (IFNγ) response elements (γIRE), and IFNγ activated sequences (GAS). These are in agreement with the gene being induced or activated *via* TNFα, IL-1, or epidermal growth factor (EGF) and the enzyme having a key regulatory role [87, 88]. Further study by the same group identified a 10 bp sequence (−17 to −8) critical for baseline expression and an AP-1 and glucocorticoid response

145

element [88]. A poly-$(CA)_{18}$ and a poly (A) polymorphism have been identified close to the 5' end of the PLA2G4 gene [85], and deletion analysis identified a functional role for the CA repeat in downregulating transcription of the gene [87]. More recently, additional forms of $cPLA_2$ have been identified, suggesting that a $cPLA_2$ family exists that is composed of three members with only modest differences in amino-acid composition; this has clear implications for regulatory mechanisms of enzyme expression and activity [89]. To date, no polymorphisms within the PLA2G4 gene have been investigated for effects on LT production or association with asthma and allergic disease.

5-Lipoxygenase (5-LO)

5-lipoxygenase is the first committed enzyme in the biosynthetic pathway leading to the production of leukotrienes and it catalyses the conversion of arachidonic acid to LTA_4. Following the isolation of cDNA from a human lung expression library, the enzyme was found to be composed of 673 amino acids with an approximate molecular weight (MW) of 85 kDa [90]. 5-LO contains essential iron and requires calcium and ATP for enzymatic activity. In agreement with a transcriptional mechanism of activation, mRNA for 5-LO at steady state is barely detectable in multiple cell lines, but following cell activation mRNA levels are elevated [56, 91]. An additional level of regulation of activity has been suggested by the requirement for translocation from the cytosol to the perinuclear membrane [92]. Increased expression of 5-LO mRNA in the peripheral blood leukocytes of asthmatics compared with normal patients has been observed, suggesting a role for transcriptional activation in the pathogenesis of asthma [93]. The importance of transcriptional activation is also supported by the paradoxical finding that dexamethasone can upregulate ALOX5 transcription in monocytes [76] and mast cells [94].

The 5-LO gene (ALOX5) has been mapped to chromosome 10q11.2 [95], spans approximately 82 kb, and is composed of 14 exons and 13 introns (Fig. 3). The 5'UTR has been characterised extensively, and one major transcription initiation site was identified 65 bp upstream of the initiation codon (ATG). Several transcription factor binding sites, including Sp1, Sp3, Egr-1, GATA-2, NK-Kap, and AP-2, were also predicted [95, 96]. The promoter region contains no TATA and CCAAT sequences, which are typically in close proximity to the transcription initiation sites of housekeeping genes [95, 96]. Within the core promoter, a GC-rich region was identified that was composed of five tandem Sp1 binding sites (–212 to –88) and was found to be essential for transcriptional activity [96]. Interestingly, alternative transcripts of ALOX5 have been described, generated by alternative splicing or transcription initiation [97].

Following mutational analysis of the ALOX5 gene, several polmorphisms were identified within the ORF and regulatory regions. These included three conservative

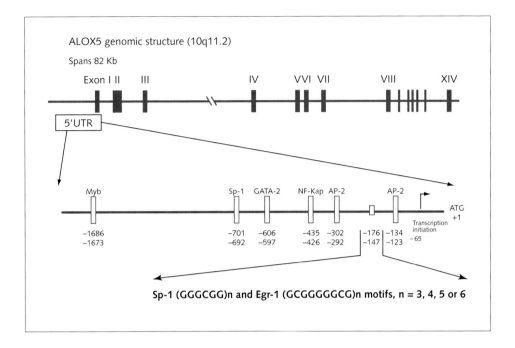

Figure 3
Schematic representation of the ALOX5 gene.
The promoter region has been enlarged and includes several potential transcription factor binding sites. The Sp1/Egr1 polymophism identified by In and co-workers [98] is illustrated. Sequence source (M38191) [96].

coding region polymorphisms (exon 1 21 C/T, exon 2 270 G/A, exon 13 1728 A/G), two promoter region polymorphisms (–1708 G/A and –1761 G/A) and a series of mutations within the G + C-rich transcription factor binding region at position –147 to –176 bp [98]. This series of mutations involved the deletion of one, deletion of two, or addition of one zinc finger (Sp1/Egr1) binding site (Fig. 3). The mutant alleles (n < or > 5) resulted in reduced Sp1/Erg1 binding and reporter gene transcription assessed by electrophoretic mobility shift assay and transient promoter-CAT transfections of HeLa cells. A reduction of 20–40% was observed when compared with the wild-type promoter [98], and specific binding of Sp1/Egr1 to the polymorphic region was confirmed in a second study by deoxyribonuclease I footprinting [99]. Using the *Drosophilia* SL2 co-transfection system, a linear relationship was identified between the number of Sp1/Egr1 motifs and transcriptional activation [99], in contrast to the initial finding in the HeLa cells. The identification of the ALOX5 Sp1/Egr1 promoter polymorphism and its subsequent functional characterisation

147

has clear implications for genetic regulation of LT production. Although only a modest change in transcriptional regulation was observed, in combination with other regulatory polymorphisms, this variant may be significant. Intriguingly, a pharmacogenetic influence for this polymorphism was identified when examining clinical responses to the 5-LO inhibitor ABT-761, as described below [100]. To date, no large-scale association study has been performed for asthma and atopy phenotypes. However, the significance of this polymorphism in asthma as a determinant of LT production is questionable because of the low frequency of "non-wild-type" alleles in asthmatics (approximately 6%) [100]. Drazen and co-workers have published comprehensive reviews of this polymorphism and its implications for asthma [101–104].

5-lipoxygenase activating protein (FLAP)

FLAP is an 18 kDa perinuclear membrane protein that, following colocalisation with $cPLA_2$, is critical for LT synthesis because of its role in presenting arachidonic acid to the active site of 5-LO (Fig. 1). The cDNA was isolated and found to encode a 162 amino acid protein [105]. The human FLAP gene (ALOX5AP) and promoter have been cloned and characterised [106]. ALOX5AP has been mapped to chromosome 13q12 using radiation hybrid mapping [107], spans > 31 kb, and is composed of five small exons and four large introns [106]. The 5' flanking region has been characterised and includes a TATA box, GRE, and AP-1 and AP-2 transcription binding sites with a predicted transcription initiation site at −74 relative to the start codon [106]. The presence of a glucocorticoid response element (GRE) is in good agreement with the role of transcriptional activation in inflammatory mechanisms. Paradoxically, the anti-inflammatory corticosteroid dexamethasone has been shown to cause FLAP gene transcription in THP-1 cells [76, 77]. Utilising a promoter-CAT reporter system, the promoter was shown to be cell-specific; cells that did not synthesise FLAP mRNA had only low (basal) levels of expression, probably because of the basic promoter elements like the TATA box. Truncations of the promoter-CAT construct identified potential enhancer regions between −337 and −644 bp of the promoter relative to the initiation codon [106].

The ALOX5AP gene is a prime candidate gene for the regulation of LT production, as the role of FLAP in the 5-LO pathway has been shown to be critical for 5-LO enzyme activity. The presence of glucocorticoid receptor motifs in the promoter links this gene product to the modulation of inflammation responses, and FLAP mRNA expression in asthmatics compared with non-asthmatics has been shown to be significantly increased [93]. Increased protein expression of FLAP has been described in blood eosinophils of mild asthmatics compared with normal subjects, and this can be mimicked *in vitro* by treatment of normal blood eosinophils with IL-5 leading to increased cys-LT production [61].

No polymorphisms have been identified in the ALOX5AP promoter, but a rare silent polymorphism within exon 5 involving a 497 A/G substitution [108] and a common HindIII RFLP polymorphism involving a C/T substitution in intron II have been described [106]. Clearly, it is unlikely that these polymorphisms will influence gene activity and/or transcriptional activation. To date, no genetic association with LT production or asthma/atopy phenotypes has been explored for polymorphic sites within the ALOX5AP gene.

Leukotriene C_4 synthase (LTC$_4$S)

Leukotriene C_4 synthase is an 18 kDa integral membrane protein that conjugates glutathione with LTA$_4$ to form LTC$_4$, the first cysteinyl-leukotriene in the 5-LO pathway. Following the cloning of the cDNA from a COS cell/KG-1 DNA library [109] and a THP-1 cell library [110], LTC$_4$ synthase was found to have a 450 bp ORF with a deduced composition of 150 amino acids, including two consensus protein kinase C (PKC) phosphorylation sites and an N-glycosylation site. Homology analysis of LTC$_4$ synthase cDNA and protein sequence with other families of glutathione-S-transferases (GST) revealed no relationships; however, LTC$_4$ synthase showed 31% homology to FLAP and can be inhibited by the FLAP antagonist MK-886 at high concentrations, suggesting a common ancestry and a unique protein family [109]. This family has been extended to include microsomal glutothione S-transferase II (GST-II), which also can utilise LTA$_4$ as a substrate to generate LTC$_4$ [111].

The human LTC$_4$ synthase gene (LTC$_4$S) consists of 5 exons, ranging between 71 and 257 bp in size, similar to ALOX5AP, and 4 introns. The gene spans 2.51 kb (in contrast to ALOX5AP, which spans > 31 kb) and has been mapped to chromosome 5q35 [73, 112], close to the 5q31-33 chromosomal region linked to asthma and atopy phenotypes [81]. 5' extension analysis of KG-1 mRNA revealed three putative transcription initiation sites at positions –96, -69, and –66 relative to the initiation codon; intriguingly, in the monocytic cell line THP-1, a single transcription initiation site was identified at position –78 relative to the initiation codon [73] (Fig. 4).

Multiple transcription factor binding sites have been identified within the 5'UTR of LTC4S, including sites for Sp1, AP-1, AP-2, and GATA-1 [73], consistent with the induction of LTC$_4$S by PMA. Recently, there has been extensive interest in the elucidation of transcriptional regulation of this gene, and multiple transcription factors have been identified as being critical. A role for the Inr (initiator like) (–66 to –62), Sp1 (–120 to –115), and Kuppel-like (–149 to –135) transcription factors has been identified using transient transfection of luciferase constructs in THP-1 and Drosophilia SL2 cells [113]. A differential role of these transcription factor binding sites was identified in basal and cell-specific transcription, with

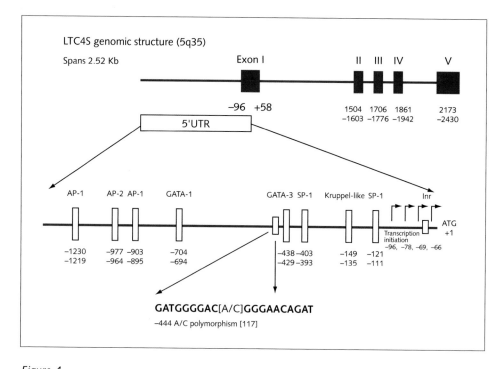

Figure 4
Schematic representation of the LTC4S gene.
The promoter region has been enlarged, illustrating several potential transcription factor binding sites including the recently described Kruppel-like site suggested to confer cell specific transcription [113]. The −444 A/C polymorphism identified by Sanak and co-workers [117] is also shown. Sequence source (U50136) [73].

the Inr and Sp1 providing basal activity and the cis-acting Kruppel-like element conferring cell specificity [113]. Transcriptional regulation of the LTC_4S gene by several agonists has been described; dexamethasone-augmented DMSO-induced transcription [114] and dexamethasone alone were shown to have no effect on transcription [94]. In addition, the cytokines TGFβ and IL-5 activate transcription, GM-CSF and IL-3 repress transcription [115], and LPS has been shown to induce transcription [116].

LTC_4S is a candidate gene for a specific subset of asthma, aspirin-intolerant asthma (AIA). These patients experience cys-LT-dependent adverse respiratory reactions to aspirin and other cyclooxygenase (COX) inhibitors, and these are superimposed upon chronically elevated cys-LT production associated with persistent severe asthma. A 5-fold over-expression of LTC_4 synthase in bronchial biopsies of AIA patients compared with ATA patients has been demonstrated, with no significant differences in other enzymes involved in the biosynthesis of cys-LTs [28]. A −444 A/C poly-morphism identified in the LTC_4 synthase gene promoter region predicts the cre-ation of an extra recognition site for the AP-2 transcription factor (Fig. 4) that may lead to enhanced gene transcription [117]. AIA patients with two variant C-444 alleles excrete more urinary LTE_4 following aspirin challenge than do AIA patients with one variant allele. Genotyping by RFLP analysis showed a doubled frequency of the variant allele in AIA patients compared with ATA or normal subjects (odds ratio 3.89) [117]. The role of the −444 LTC_4S polymorphism in AIA is controver-sial, with multiple studies from the Krakow group showing a positive association with AIA [117–119], while other groups have failed to confirm this in other popu-lations of AIA patients [108]. In a small study, we examined the role of the −444 polymorphism in severe asthmatics; the C allele (C/C and C/T) was found to be more prevalent in severe asthmatics (56%) compared with normal subjects (32%, $p = 0.04$). Compared with wild-type (AA) controls, the presence of the C allele resulted in an approximate 3-fold increase in LTC_4 production in isolated blood eosinophils stimulated with calcium ionophore A23187 in the presence of indomethacin ($p = 0.04$) [120].

The role of LTC_4S polymorphisms in determining LT production remains unclear, but accumulating evidence suggests that the −444 C allele has a role in acti-vating gene transcription. The implications of this phenomenon need to be explored in AIA.

Leukotriene A_4 hydrolase (LTA_4H)

LTA_4 hydrolase catalyses the conversion of LTA_4 to LTB_4. The enzyme is thought to be a bifunctional zinc metalloenzyme with aminopeptidase and epoxide hydrolase activity. The protein is predicted to be 69 kDa in size, and a cDNA has been cloned identifying an ORF of 1833 bp encoding 610 amino acids [121, 122]. Following the isolation of a genomic clone [123], the gene was found to span 35 kb and to con-tain 19 exons ranging in size from 24 to 312 bp, and it was mapped to chromosome 12q22 by *in situ* hybridisation. The promoter region does not contain a putative TATA box but contains multiple transcription factor binding sites including AP-2 and XREs consistent with an inducible promoter. The transcription initiation site has been mapped to −151 bp relative to the initiation codon [123]. To date, tran-scriptional regulation of the LTA_4H gene has not been investigated; the finding that LTA_4H mRNA is alternatively spliced [124] suggests that regulation is post-tran-scriptional, although this has not been investigated further. The alternative splice variants are generated by the skipping of an 83 bp exon located in the 3' coding region resulting in a protein of 59 kDa with a distinct C-terminus [124].

To date, only one mutational analysis study of the LTA_4H gene has been com-pleted [108]; 102 G/T and 114 C/T substitutions were identified in exon I, neither leading to an amino acid change. These polymorphisms are therefore unlikely to have any significant role in the regulation of leuktriene production and in asthma.

Glutamyl transpeptidase/dipeptidase

γ-glutamyltranspeptidase acts as a glutathionase and catalyses the conversion of LTC_4 to LTD_4 by cleaving the glutamic acid moiety (Fig. 1). The enzyme is found on the outer surface of the cell membrane and is widely distributed in mammalian cells. The GGT gene has been mapped to chromosome 22q11.1-11.2 [125] and the gene has been characterised [126]. It is composed of an ORF of 1709 bp encoding for the two peptide subunits of the enzyme (351 and 189 amino acids). A family of at least four GGT genes exists on chromosome 22 and at least two are transcribed [127]. To date, the genes have not been further characterised.

Dipeptidase (previously referred to as renal dipeptidase/dehydropeptidase I) is a kidney membrane enzyme that has been implicated in the hydrolysis of glutathione and its conjugates, including LTD_4 [128]. It is a key enzyme in the production of LTE_4, the final cys-LT in the 5-LO pathway. A cDNA clone of the gene (DPEP1) has been identified [129], which has been mapped to chromosome 16p24.3. To date, the gene has not been further characterised.

Intriguingly, in a GGT-deficient mouse, the ability to convert LTC_4 to LTD_4 was retained, suggesting a role for an additional enzyme termed γ-glutamyl leukotrienase (GGL) [130]. Similarly, mice deficient in membrane-bound dipeptidase retained the ability to convert LTD_4 to LTE_4, again suggesting the involvement of multiple enzymes [131]. Clearly, clarification of the enzymology is required prior to a detailed genetic analysis.

Molecular biology of LT receptors

LTB_4 receptor (BLT)

As described above, the proinflammatory actions of LTB_4 are mediated by the G-protein coupled receptor BLT. The cDNA for BLT was isolated independently by two groups [132, 133] (designated CMKRL1 and P2Y7 since the ligand was not identified at this time). The cDNA encodes a 352 amino acid polypeptide with a calculated MW of 43 kDa, which was predicted to have seven putative transmembrane domains. The sequence showed homology to the chemoattractant leukocyte receptors, including C5a anaphylatoxin receptor. Transcripts were identified in several tissues including the spleen, thymus, and lymph node, suggesting an inflammatory role [132], and in the human heart, skeletal muscle, brain, and liver [133]. Two cDNA clones (1.5 and 3.0 kb mRNA species) were isolated from HL-60 cells that contained identical ORF (seven membrane spanning domains) but had different 5' untranslated regions [134]. Transfection studies using CHO cells confirmed that the receptor was BLT and not a purinoceptor [134].

The human BLT gene has been mapped to chromosome 14q11.2-12 [132], is approximately 5 kb in size, and is composed of three exons [135]. The ORF of BLT is in exon 3, and two distinct 5'untranslated regions have been identified in exon 1 and 2 [135]. To date, no analyses of the promoter or of the contribution of genetic polymorphism within the BLT gene have been completed. Polymorphism within the BLT gene does seem possible because of the finding that other seven-transmembrane GCPR have multiple polymorphisms, e.g., the β-adrenergic receptor.

CysLT$_1$ receptor

The CysLT$_1$ receptor is critical for the activity of cys-LTs, and antagonism of this protein has been effective in the treatment of asthma. The cDNA encoding the CysLT$_1$ receptor was cloned in 1999 almost simultaneously by two independent groups [35, 36]. Both groups used the orphan GPCR approach to identify ESTs that showed homology to known GPCR followed by ligand fishing. The cDNA was found to have an ORF of 1014 bp encoding for a 337 amino-acid protein that showed 28% homology to BLT with a calculated MW of 38 kDa (Fig. 5). Transfection of the cRNA into *Xenopus leavis* oocytes identified an LTD$_4$ dose-dependent, calcium-activated chloride conductance channel with an EC$_{50}$ of 3 nM, and similar studies in melanophores identified the affinities LTD$_4$ >> LTE$_4$ = LTC$_4$ >> LTB$_4$ [35]. The CysLT$_1$ receptor antagonists MK-571, montelukast, and zarfirlukast displayed high affinity for CysLT$_1$. Transcript was identified in human lung and smooth muscle, and the gene was mapped to chromosome Xq13-21 [35]. Similar findings were reported by the second group using human embryonic kidney (HEK) cells; the recombinant receptor had affinities LTD$_4$ > LTC$_4$ > LTE$_4$, and, again, expression was identified in the human lung, bronchus, and peripheral blood leukocytes [36].

To date, no genomic sequence has been published for the CysLT$_1$ gene, but in collaboration with Merck two studies have mutation-scanned the genomic sequence. Pulleyn and co-workers identified a rare silent polymorphism in the ORF using SSCP but did not disclose the nature of the substitution or its position [136]. Bolk and co-workers identified two missense SNPs (617 T/G, 898 G/A) and one silent SNP (927 T/C) [137]. The two missense variants result in amino-acid substitutions: Ile206Ser and Gly300Ser. Residue 206 is in the fifth transmembrane domain and residue 300 is in the intracellular tail in the predicted structure of the receptor (Fig. 5). Clearly, these polymorphisms may have functional consequences, resulting in differential cys-LT activity in certain individuals. The 617 G allele and the 898 A allele were found in only 2 of the 58 chromosomes tested, indicating a low fre-

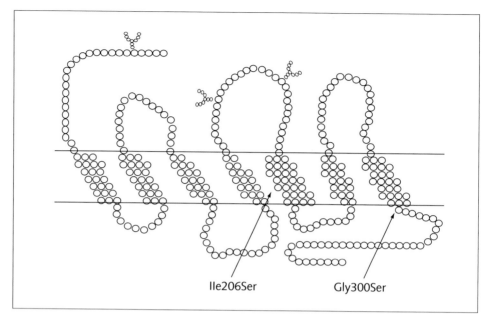

Ile206Ser   Gly300Ser

Figure 5

Representation of the CysLT_1 receptor.

The putative seven-transmembrane segments were identified based on the hydropathicity profile of the amino-acid sequence [35]. Potential glycosylation sites are illustrated, and the position of the two amino-acid substitutions resulting from two missense polymorphisms in the ORF are shown [137].

quency for both alleles (0.03). In view of the low frequency of these polymorphisms, a significant role in asthma is doubtful, although they may influence LT activity in this small subgroup of the population. Studies are ongoing in several laboratories to clarify the role of these polymorphisms.

CysLT$_2$ receptor

During the writing of this review, the cloning of the CysLT$_2$ receptor has been reported [37]. Essentially, using the same orphan GPCR approach, a cDNA encoding a 346 amino acid GPCR with 38% amino acid homology to CysLT$_1$ was identified. Transfection studies in *Xenopus* oocytes and HEK293T cells identified the affinities of LTC$_4$ = LTD$_4$ >> LTE$_4$. In contrast to the selective CysLT$_1$ antagonists MK-571, montelukast, zafirlukast, and pranlukast, only the dual CysLT$_1$/CysLT$_2$ antagonist BAY u9773 had a significant antagonistic effect on CysLT$_2$ [37]. CysLT$_2$

transcript has been identified in lung macrophages, airway smooth muscle, cardiac Purkinje cells, adrenal medulla cells, peripheral leukocytes, and the brain. The gene has been mapped to chromosome 13q14, a region linked to asthma and atopy phenotypes. The cloning of the $CysLT_2$ receptor now permits a comprehensive characterisation of the role of this receptor in LT activity and in several disorders. Intriguing evidence suggesting that cys-LTs have a role in airway remodelling in asthma *via* the interaction with multiple receptors [138] can now be assessed.

In the absence of a genomic clone for $CysLT_2$, mutational analysis of the ORF is possible using RNA and cDNA analysis, but the characterisation of regulatory regions can proceed only following the publication of the genomic sequence. The role of $CysLT_2$ is poorly understood, but polymorphism within the gene may have significant implications for LT activity and diseases such as asthma.

Pharmacogenetics of LT modifier drugs

As described previously, LT modifier drugs have shown clinical efficiency over a wide spectrum of asthma severity. The distribution of clinical responsiveness to LTRA is controversial. Some studies and anecdotal clinical evidence suggest that a minority of patients respond extremely well to LTRAs (approximately 10–15%), with a large subgroup (approximately 50%) showing a significant clinical improvement and a minority not responding at all. However, a large clinical trial suggests a continuous bell-shaped distribution of response to montelukast that parallels responses to the inhaled corticosteroid beclomethasone [139]. Nevertheless, the heterogeneity of response observed with leukotriene modifier drugs may have a genetic basis, and the identification of genetically determined "responder" and "nonresponder" phenotypes might be clinically useful and lead to fundamental insights into differential disease mechanisms.

In a small study of poorly controlled severe asthmatics, we examined the pharmacogenetic influence of the LTC4S –444 polymorphism on response to an LT modifier drug. The response to two weeks of treatment with zafirlukast (Accolate 20 mg bd) depended on genotype, with FEV_1 increasing by 9 ± 12% in individuals with the C allele and decreasing by –12 ± 18% in the AA genotype group [120].

Drazen and co-workers have examined the role of the ALOX5 Sp1/Egr1 polymorphism in the pharmacogenetics of LT modifier drugs. In 221 asthmatics, those possesing only mutant ALOX5 alleles were relatively resistant to treatment with the LT synthesis inhibitor ABT-761. Mean FEV_1 improved by approximately 18.8 ± 3.6% (n = 64) for WT homozygotes and 23.3 ± 6% (n = 40) for heterozygotes, compared with –1.2 ± 2.9% (n = 10) in homozygote mutant individuals [100].

The concepts demonstrated by these two studies are simple in nature: genetic predisposition to over-production of LT results in the expression of an asthma phenotype that is more dependent on LT production. These patients respond better to drugs that target these mediators because leukotriene production is central to the pathogenic mechanisms in this form of asthma, while other mediators may play a more important role in other asthmatic patients.

Conclusions and future prospects

This review has presented accumulating evidence that polymorphism within the genes that regulate LT production or activity may have a significant role in the predisposition to specific asthma phenotypes and in clinical responsiveness to LT modifier drugs. LTC_4S and ALOX5 promoter polymorphisms have been the focus of much attention and have been shown to influence LT production and to identify individuals that have a "leukotriene-dependent" phenotype of asthma. These individuals may be more responsive to LT modifier therapy.

A subset of asthmatics in whom leukotrienes are the major contributory factor in causing allergic inflammation has recently been described in a study designed to determine the effects of allergen exposure on LT production in BAL fluid in the presence and absence of the 5-LO inhibitor zileuton [140]. The study identified distinct sub-groups of high and low cys-LT producers following allergen challenge; zileuton was effective in reducing eosinophil counts in the high LT producers compared with no detectable effect in the low producers [140]. The high LT producers also had significantly higher BAL fluid levels of LTB_4 and of a range of pro-inflammatory and Th2-type cytokines. The study is the first to link clinical responses to a LT modifier drug to excess LT production in the lung and to a specific cellular phenotype, specifically to airway eosinophilia. Genetic predisposition is obviously one potential explanation for the subsets of patients observed in this study. Support for "leukotriene-dependent" inflammation being genetically determined has recently been derived from studies of different strains of 5-LO-deficient mice [141]. Using an arachidonic acid-induced inflammation model, mouse strains 129 and DBA were found to have LT-mediated inflammation, whereas B6 mice were found to have inflammation independent of LT but dependent on prostanoids [141].

Clearly, more work is required in order to further the understanding of the regulation of the genes involved in LT synthesis and activity before conclusions can be made, but studies in both the human and mouse suggest a genetic predisposition to a leukotriene-dependent phenotype. The recent cloning of the $CysLT_1$ and $CysLT_2$ receptors has now made possible the investigation of genetic predisposition to variable receptor responses to LTs and to LT modifier drugs. Indeed, multiple polymorphisms within the $CysLT_1$ receptor have been identified and are being investigated in several laboratories worldwide.

In simplistic terms, asthma is predicted to involve multiple genetic polymorphisms, including variations in LT synthesis and activity, which together constitute a heterogeneous genetic background, but this is expressed only phenotypically in the presence of multiple environmental triggers. Pharmacogenetic targeting of LT modifier drugs to those patients most likely to respond is one potential benefit from these studies. However, the true value of a better understanding of the genetic basis of LT production and activity will be the fundamental insights gained into the heterogeneity of mechanisms underlying asthma pathogenesis.

References

1   Holgate S, Dahlen S-E (eds) (1997) *SRS-A to leukotrienes: The dawning of a new treatment*. Blackwell Science, Oxford, UK, 336

2   Drazen JM, Israel E, O'Byrne PM (1999) Treatment of asthma with drugs modifying the leukotriene pathway [published errata appear in *N Engl J Med* (1999) 340 (8): 663 and 341 (21): 1632]. *N Engl J Med* 340: 197–206

3   Holgate ST, Sampson AP (2000) Antileukotriene therapy. Future directions. *Am J Respir Crit Care Med* 161: S147–153

4   Samuelsson B (1987) An elucidation of the arachidonic acid cascade. Discovery of prostaglandins, thromboxane and leukotrienes. *Drugs* 33 (Suppl 1): 2–9

5   MacGlashan DW, Jr., Schleimer RP, Peters SP, Schulman ES, Adams GKd, Newball HH, Lichtenstein LM (1982) Generation of leukotrienes by purified human lung mast cells. *J Clin Invest* 70: 747–751

6   Weller PF, Lee CW, Foster DW, Corey EJ, Austen KF, Lewis RA (1983) Generation and metabolism of 5-lipoxygenase pathway leukotrienes by human eosinophils: Predominant production of leukotriene c4. *Proc Natl Acad Sci USA* 80: 7626–7630

7   Williams JD, Czop JK, Austen KF (1984) Release of leukotrienes by human monocytes on stimulation of their phagocytic receptor for particulate activators. *J Immunol* 132: 3034–3040

8   Dahlen SE, Hedqvist P, Hammarstrom S, Samuelsson B (1980) Leukotrienes are potent constrictors of human bronchi. *Nature* 288: 484–486

9   Weiss JW, Drazen JM, McFadden ER Jr, Weller P, Corey EJ, Lewis RA, Austen KF (1983) Airway constriction in normal humans produced by inhalation of leukotriene d. Potency, time course, and effect of aspirin therapy. *Jama* 249: 2814–2817

10   Barnes NC, Piper PJ, Costello JF (1984) Comparative effects of inhaled leukotriene c4, leukotriene d4, and histamine in normal human subjects. *Thorax* 39: 500–504

11   Marom Z, Shelhamer JH, Bach MK, Morton DR, Kaliner M (1982) Slow-reacting substances, leukotrienes c4 and d4, increase the release of mucus from human airways *in vitro*. *Am Rev Respir Dis* 126: 449–451

12   Arm JP, Lee TH (1993) Sulphidopeptide leukotrienes in asthma [editorial]. *Clin Sci (Colch)* 84: 501–510

13   Bousquet J, Chanez P, Lacoste JY, Barneon G, Ghavanian N, Enander I, Venge P, Ahlstedt S, Simony-Lafontaine J, Godard P et al (1990) Eosinophilic inflammation in asthma. *N Engl J Med* 323: 1033–1039

14 Laitinen LA, Laitinen A, Haahtela T, Vilkka V, Spur BW, Lee TH (1993) Leukotriene e4 and granulocytic infiltration into asthmatic airways. *Lancet* 341: 989–990

15 Spada CS, Nieves AL, Krauss AH, Woodward DF (1994) Comparison of leukotriene b4 and d4 effects on human eosinophil and neutrophil motility *in vitro*. *J Leukoc Biol* 55: 183–191

16 Okubo T, Takahashi H, Sumitomo M, Shindoh K, Suzuki S (1987) Plasma levels of leukotrienes c4 and d4 during wheezing attack in asthmatic patients. *Int Arch Allergy Appl Immunol* 84: 149–155

17 Wenzel SE, Larsen GL, Johnston K, Voelkel NF, Westcott JY (1990) Elevated levels of leukotriene c4 in bronchoalveolar lavage fluid from atopic asthmatics after endobronchial allergen challenge. *Am Rev Respir Dis* 142: 112–119

18 Taylor GW, Taylor I, Black P, Maltby NH, Turner N, Fuller RW, Dollery CT (1989) Urinary leukotriene e4 after antigen challenge and in acute asthma and allergic rhinitis. *Lancet* 1: 584–588

19 Kumlin M, Dahlen B, Bjorck T, Zetterstrom O, Granstrom E, Dahlen SE (1992) Urinary excretion of leukotriene e4 and 11-dehydro-thromboxane b2 in response to bronchial provocations with allergen, aspirin, leukotriene d4, and histamine in asthmatics. *Am Rev Respir Dis* 146: 96–103

20 Ferreri NR, Howland WC, Stevenson DD, Spiegelberg HL (1988) Release of leukotrienes, prostaglandins, and histamine into nasal secretions of aspirin-sensitive asthmatics during reaction to aspirin. *Am Rev Respir Dis* 137: 847–854

21 Picado C, Ramis I, Rosello J, Prat J, Bulbena O, Plaza V, Montserrat JM, Gelpi E (1992) Release of peptide leukotriene into nasal secretions after local instillation of aspirin in aspirin-sensitive asthmatic patients. *Am Rev Respir Dis* 145: 65–69

22 Creticos PS, Peters SP, Adkinson NF, Jr., Naclerio RM, Hayes EC, Norman PS, Lichtenstein LM (1984) Peptide leukotriene release after antigen challenge in patients sensitive to ragweed. *N Engl J Med* 310: 1626–1630

23 Hoover RL, Karnovsky MJ, Austen KF, Corey EJ, Lewis RA (1984) Leukotriene b4 action on endothelium mediates augmented neutrophil/endothelial adhesion. *Proc Natl Acad Sci USA* 81: 2191–2193

24 Yamaoka KA, Kolb JP (1993) Leukotriene b4 induces interleukin 5 generation from human t lymphocytes. *Eur J Immunol* 23: 2392–2398

25 Brach MA, de Vos S, Arnold C, Gruss HJ, Mertelsmann R, Herrmann F (1992) Leukotriene b4 transcriptionally activates interleukin-6 expression involving nk-chi b and nf-il6. *Eur J Immunol* 22: 2705–2711

26 Devchand PR, Keller H, Peters JM, Vazquez M, Gonzalez FJ, Wahli W (1996) The ppa-ralpha-leukotriene b4 pathway to inflammation control. *Nature* 384: 39–43

27 Aoki Y, Qiu D, Zhao GH, Kao PN (1998) Leukotriene b4 mediates histamine induction of nf-kappab and il-8 in human bronchial epithelial cells. *Am J Physiol* 274: L1030–1039

28 Cowburn AS, Sladek K, Soja J, Adamek L, Nizankowska E, Szczeklik A, Lam BK, Penrose JF, Austen FK, Holgate ST et al (1998) Overexpression of leukotriene c4 synthase

in bronchial biopsies from patients with aspirin-intolerant asthma. *J Clin Invest* 101: 834–846

29 Dahlen SE, Haeggstrom JZ, Samuelsson B, Rabe KF, Leff AR (2000) Leukotrienes as targets for the treatment of asthma and other diseases: Current basic and clinical research. *Am J Crit Care Med* 161 (Suppl): S1–153

30 Coleman RA, Eglen RM, Jones RL, Narumiya S, Shimizu T, Smith WL, Dahlen SE, Drazen JM, Gardiner PJ, Jackson WT et al (1995) Prostanoid and leukotriene receptors: A progress report from the iuphar working parties on classification and nomenclature. *Adv Prostaglandin Thromboxane Leukot Res* 23: 283–285

31 Metters KM (1995) Leukotriene receptors. *J Lipid Mediat Cell Signal* 12: 413–427

32 Votta B, Mong S (1990) Transition of affinity states for leukotriene b4 receptors in sheep lung membranes. *Biochem J* 265: 841–847

33 Owman C, Sabirsh A, Garzino-Demo A, Cocchi F (2000) Cloning of a novel chemoattractant receptor activated by leukotriene b4 and used by human immunodeficiency virus type 1 to infect cd4-positive immune cells. A therapeutic connection to asthma? *Am J Respir Crit Care Med* 161: S56–61

34 Labat C, Ortiz JL, Norel X, Gorenne I, Verley J, Abram TS, Cuthbert NJ, Tudhope SR, Norman P, Gardiner P et al (1992) A second cysteinyl leukotriene receptor in human lung. *J Pharmacol Exp Ther* 263: 800–805

35 Lynch KR, O'Neill GP, Liu Q, Im DS, Sawyer N, Metters KM, Coulombe N, Abramovitz M, Figueroa DJ, Zeng Z et al (1999) Characterization of the human cysteinyl leukotriene cyslt1 receptor. *Nature* 399: 789–793

36 Sarau HM, Ames RS, Chambers J, Ellis C, Elshourbagy N, Foley JJ, Schmidt DB, Muccitelli RM, Jenkins O, Murdock PR et al (1999) Identification, molecular cloning, expression, and characterization of a cysteinyl leukotriene receptor. *Mol Pharmacol* 56: 657–663

37 Heise CE, O'Dowd BF, Figueroa DJ, Sawyer N, Nguyen T, Im DS, Stocco R, Bellefeuille JN, Abramovitz M, Cheng R et al (2000) Characterization of the human cysteinyl leukotriene 2 (CysLT$_2$) receptor. *J Biol Chem* 275: 30531–30536

38 Sampson A, Holgate S (1998) Leukotriene modifiers in the treatment of asthma. Look promising across the board of asthma severity [editorial]. *BMJ* 316: 1257–1258

39 Holgate ST, Bradding P, Sampson AP (1996) Leukotriene antagonists and synthesis inhibitors: New directions in asthma therapy. *J Allergy Clin Immunol* 98: 1–13

40 Spector SL, Smith LJ, Glass M (1994) Effects of 6 weeks of therapy with oral doses of ici 204,219, a leukotriene d4 receptor antagonist, in subjects with bronchial asthma. Accolate asthma trialists group. *Am J Respir Crit Care Med* 150: 618–623

41 Evans DJ, Barnes PJ, Spaethe SM, van Alstyne EL, Mitchell MI, O'Connor BJ (1996) Effect of a leukotriene b4 receptor antagonist, ly293111, on allergen induced responses in asthma. *Thorax* 51: 1178–1184

42 Seymour M, Aberg D, Riise G, Rak S, Holgate S, Sampson A (1998) Seasonal allergen exposure increases expression of leukotriene pathway enzymes and induces eosinophil influx in bronchial mucosa of atopic asthmatics. *J Allergy Clin Immunol* 101: 711 (abstr)

43 Taniguchi N, Mita H, Saito H, Yui Y, Kajita T, Shida T (1985) Increased generation of leukotriene c4 from eosinophils in asthmatic patients. *Allergy* 40: 571–573

44 Bruijnzeel PL, Virchow JC, Jr., Rihs S, Walker C, Verhagen J (1993) Lack of increased numbers of low-density eosinophils in the circulation of asthmatic individuals. *Clin Exp Allergy* 23: 261–269

45 Laviolette M, Ferland C, Comtois JF, Champagne K, Bosse M, Boulet LP (1995) Blood eosinophil leukotriene c4 production in asthma of different severities. *Eur Respir J* 8: 1465–1472

46 Silberstein DS, Owen WF, Gasson JC, DiPersio JF, Golde DW, Bina JC, Soberman R, Austen KF, David JR (1986) Enhancement of human eosinophil cytotoxicity and leukotriene synthesis by biosynthetic (recombinant) granulocyte-macrophage colony-stimulating factor. *J Immunol* 137: 3290–3294

47 Rothenberg ME, Owen WF, Jr., Silberstein DS, Woods J, Soberman RJ, Austen KF, Stevens RL (1988) Human eosinophils have prolonged survival, enhanced functional properties, and become hypodense when exposed to human interleukin 3. *J Clin Invest* 81: 1986–1992

48 Rothenberg ME, Petersen J, Stevens RL, Silberstein DS, McKenzie DT, Austen KF, Owen WF Jr (1989) Il-5-dependent conversion of normodense human eosinophils to the hypo-dense phenotype uses 3t3 fibroblasts for enhanced viability, accelerated hypodensity, and sustained antibody-dependent cytotoxicity. *J Immunol* 143: 2311–2316

49 Takafuji S, Bischoff SC, De Weck AL, Dahinden CA (1991) Il-3 and il-5 prime normal human eosinophils to produce leukotriene c4 in response to soluble agonists. *J Immunol* 147: 3855–3861

50 Boyce JA, Lam BK, Penrose JF, Friend DS, Parsons S, Owen WF, Austen KF (1996) Expression of ltc4 synthase during the development of eosinophils *in vitro* from cord blood progenitors. *Blood* 88: 4338–4347

51 DiPersio JF, Billing P, Williams R, Gasson JC (1988) Human granulocyte-macrophage colony-stimulating factor and other cytokines prime human neutrophils for enhanced arachidonic acid release and leukotriene b4 synthesis. *J Immunol* 140: 4315–4322

52 McColl SR, DiPersio JF, Caon AC, Ho P, Naccache PH (1991) Involvement of tyrosine kinases in the activation of human peripheral blood neutrophils by granulocyte-macrophage colony-stimulating factor. *Blood* 78: 1842–1852

53 Pouliot M, McDonald PP, Khamzina L, Borgeat P, McColl SR (1994) Granulocyte-macrophage colony-stimulating factor enhances 5-lipoxygenase levels in human poly-morphonuclear leukocytes. *J Immunol* 152: 851–858

54 Pouliot M, McDonald PP, Borgeat P, McColl SR (1994) Granulocyte/macrophage colony-stimulating factor stimulates the expression of the 5-lipoxygenase-activating pro-tein (flap) in human neutrophils. *J Exp Med* 179: 1225–1232

55 Stankova J, Rola-Pleszczynski M, Dubois CM (1995) Granulocyte-macrophage colony-stimulating factor increases 5-lipoxygenase gene transcription and protein expression in human neutrophils. *Blood* 85: 3719–3726

56 Ring WL, Riddick CA, Baker JR, Munafo DA, Bigby TD (1996) Lymphocytes stimulate

expression of 5-lipoxygenase and its activating protein in monocytes *in vitro via* granulocyte macrophage colony-stimulating factor and interleukin 3. *J Clin Invest* 97: 1293–1301

57   Ring WL, Riddick CA, Baker JR, Glass CK, Bigby TD (1997) Activated lymphocytes increase expression of 5-lipoxygenase and its activating protein in thp-1 cells. *Am J Physiol* 273: C2057–2064

58   Bennett CF, Chiang MY, Monia BP, Crooke ST (1993) Regulation of 5-lipoxygenase and 5-lipoxygenase-activating protein expression in hl-60 cells. *Biochem J* 289: 33–39

59   Brungs M, Radmark O, Samuelsson B, Steinhilber D (1995) Sequential induction of 5-lipoxygenase gene expression and activity in mono mac 6 cells by transforming growth factor beta and 1,25-dihydroxyvitamin d3. *Proc Natl Acad Sci USA* 92: 107–111

60   Nassar GM, Montero A, Fukunaga M, Badr KF (1997) Contrasting effects of proinflammatory and t-helper lymphocyte subset-2 cytokines on the 5-lipoxygenase pathway in monocytes. *Kidney Int* 51: 1520–1528

61   Cowburn AS, Holgate ST, Sampson AP (1999) Il-5 increases expression of 5-lipoxygenase-activating protein and translocates 5-lipoxygenase to the nucleus in human blood eosinophils. *J Immunol* 163: 456–465

62   Coffey MJ, Wilcoxen SE, Peters-Golden M (1994) Increases in 5-lipoxygenase activating protein expression account for enhanced capacity for 5-lipoxygenase metabolism that accompanies differentiation of peripheral blood monocytes into alveolar macrophages. *Am J Respir Cell Mol Biol* 11: 153–158

63   Bradding P, Roberts JA, Britten KM, Montefort S, Djukanovic R, Mueller R, Heusser CH, Howarth PH, Holgate ST (1994) Interleukin-4, -5, and -6 and tumor necrosis factor-alpha in normal and asthmatic airways: Evidence for the human mast cell as a source of these cytokines. *Am J Respir Cell Mol Biol* 10: 471–480

64   Corrigan CJ, Haczku A, Gemou-Engesaeth V, Doi S, Kikuchi Y, Takatsu K, Durham SR, Kay AB (1993) Cd4 t-lymphocyte activation in asthma is accompanied by increased serum concentrations of interleukin-5. Effect of glucocorticoid therapy. *Am Rev Respir Dis* 147: 540–547

65   Brown PH, Crompton GK, Greening AP (1991) Proinflammatory cytokines in acute asthma. *Lancet* 338: 590–593

65a   Miyajima A, Mui AL, Ogorochi T, Sakamaki K (1993) Receptors for granulocyte colony-stimulating factor, interleukin 3, and interleukin 5. *Blood* 82 (7): 1960–1974

66   van der Bruggen T, Caldenhoven E, Kanters D, Coffer P, Raaijmakers JA, Lammers JW, Koenderman L (1995) Interleukin-5 signaling in human eosinophils involves jak2 tyrosine kinase and stat1 alpha. *Blood* 85: 1442–1448

67   van der Bruggen T, Kanters D, Tool AT, Raaijmakers JA, Lammers JW, Verhoeven AJ, Koenderman L (1998) Cytokine-induced protein tyrosine phosphorylation is essential for cytokine priming of human eosinophils. *J Allergy Clin Immunol* 101: 103–109

68   Woods JW, Evans JF, Ethier D, Scott S, Vickers PJ, Hearn L, Heibein JA, Charleson S, Singer, II (1993) 5-lipoxygenase and 5-lipoxygenase-activating protein are localized in the nuclear envelope of activated human leukocytes. *J Exp Med* 178: 1935–1946

69 Brock TG, McNish RW, Bailie MB, Peters-Golden M (1997) Rapid import of cytosolic 5-lipoxygenase into the nucleus of neutrophils after *in vivo* recruitment and *in vitro* adherence. *J Biol Chem* 272: 8276–8280

70 Brock TG, Anderson JA, Fries FP, Peters-Golden M, Sporn PH (1999) Decreased leukotriene c4 synthesis accompanies adherence-dependent nuclear import of 5-lipoxygenase in human blood eosinophils. *J Immunol* 162: 1669–1676

71 Lepley RA, Fitzpatrick FA (1994) 5-lipoxygenase contains a functional src homology 3-binding motif that interacts with the src homology 3 domain of grb2 and cytoskeletal proteins. *J Biol Chem* 269: 24163–24168

72 Lepley RA, Muskardin DT, Fitzpatrick FA (1996) Tyrosine kinase activity modulates catalysis and translocation of cellular 5-lipoxygenase. *J Biol Chem* 271: 6179–6184

73 Penrose JF, Spector J, Baldasaro M, Xu K, Boyce J, Arm JP, Austen KF, Lam BK (1996) Molecular cloning of the gene for human leukotriene c4 synthase. Organization, nucleotide sequence, and chromosomal localization to 5q35. *J Biol Chem* 271: 11356–11361

74 Peers SH, Flower RJ (1990) The role of lipocortin in corticosteroid actions. *Am Rev Respir Dis* 141: S18–21

75 Djukanovic R, Wilson JW, Britten KM, Wilson SJ, Walls AF, Roche WR, Howarth PH, Holgate ST (1992) Effect of an inhaled corticosteroid on airway inflammation and symptoms in asthma. *Am Rev Respir Dis* 145: 669–674

76 Riddick CA, Ring WL, Baker JR, Hodulik CR, Bigby TD (1997) Dexamethasone increases expression of 5-lipoxygenase and its activating protein in human monocytes and thp-1 cells. *Eur J Biochem* 246: 112–118

77 Goppelt-Struebe M, Schaefer D, Habenicht AJ (1997) Differential regulation of cyclooxygenase-2 and 5-lipoxygenase-activating protein (flap) expression by glucocorticoids in monocytic cells. *Br J Pharmacol* 122: 619–624

78 Scoggan KA, Ford-Hutchinson AW, Nicholson DW (1995) Differential activation of leukotriene biosynthesis by granulocyte-macrophage colony-stimulating factor and interleukin-5 in an eosinophilic substrain of hl-60 cells. *Blood* 86: 3507–3516

79 Manso G, Baker AJ, Taylor IK, Fuller RW (1992) *In vivo* and *in vitro* effects of glucocorticosteroids on arachidonic acid metabolism and monocyte function in nonasthmatic humans. *Eur Respir J* 5: 712–716

80 Dworski R, Fitzgerald GA, Oates JA, Sheller JR (1994) Effect of oral prednisone on airway inflammatory mediators in atopic asthma. *Am J Respir Crit Care Med* 149: 953–959

81 Sayers I, Beghe B, Holloway J, Holgate S (2000) Genetics of asthma: What's new? In: SHS Johnston (ed): *Challenges in asthma*. Blackwell Science, Oxford, UK, 138–168

82 Shamsuddin M, Chen E, Anderson J, Smith LJ (1997) Regulation of leukotriene and platelet-activating factor synthesis in human alveolar macrophages. *J Lab Clin Med* 130: 615–626

83 Uozumi N, Kume K, Nagase T, Nakatani N, Ishii S, Tashiro F, Komagata Y, Maki K, Ikuta K, Ouchi Y et al (1997) Role of cytosolic phospholipase A2 in allergic response and parturition. *Nature* 390: 618–622

84 Peters-Golden M, McNish RW (1993) Redistribution of 5-lipoxygenase and cytosolic phospholipase a2 to the nuclear fraction upon macrophage activation. *Biochem Biophys Res Commun* 196: 147–153

85 Tay A, Simon JS, Squire J, Hamel K, Jacob HJ, Skorecki K (1995) Cytosolic phospholipase a2 gene in human and rat: Chromosomal localization and polymorphic markers. *Genomics* 26: 138–141

86 Sharp J, White D, G Chiou (1991) Molecular cloning and expression of human ca(2+)-sensitive cytosolic phospholipase a2. *J Biol Chem* 266: 14850–14853

87 Wu T, Ikezono T, Angus W, Shelhamer J (1994) Characterisation of the promoter of the human 85 kda cytosolic phospholipase a2 gene. *Nucleic Acid Research* 22: 5093–5098

88 Miyashita A, Crystal RG, Hay JG (1995) Identification of a 27 bp 5'-flanking region element responsible for the low level constitutive expression of the human cytosolic phospholipase a2 gene. *Nucleic Acids Res* 23: 293–301

89 Song C, Chang XJ, Bean KM, Proia MS, Knopf JL, Kriz RW (1999) Molecular characterization of cytosolic phospholipase a2-beta. *J Biol Chem* 274: 17063–17067

90 Matsumoto T, Funk CD, Radmark O, Hoog JO, Jornvall H, Samuelsson B (1988) Molecular cloning and amino acid sequence of human 5-lipoxygenase [published erratum appears in Proc Natl Acad Sci USA (1988) 85 (10): 3406]. *Proc Natl Acad Sci USA* 85: 26–30

91 Steinhilber D, Brungs M, Radmark O, Samuelsson B (1995) Transforming growth factor-beta and 1,25-dihydroxyvitamin d3 induce 5-lipoxygenase activity during myeloid cell maturation. *Adv Prostaglandin Thromboxane Leukot Res* 23: 449–451

92 Coffey M, Peters-Golden M, Fantone JCd, Sporn PH (1992) Membrane association of active 5-lipoxygenase in resting cells. Evidence for novel regulation of the enzyme in the rat alveolar macrophage. *J Biol Chem* 267: 570–576

93 Koshino T, Takano S, Houjo T, Sano Y, Kudo K, Kihara H, Kitani S, Takaishi T, Hirai K, Ito K et al (1998) Expression of 5-lipoxygenase and 5-lipoxygenase-activating protein mrnas in the peripheral blood leukocytes of asthmatics. *Biochem Biophys Res Commun* 247: 510–513

94 Colamorea T, Di Paola R, Macchia F, Guerrese MC, Tursi A, Butterfield JH, Caiaffa MF, Haeggstrom JZ, Macchia L (1999) 5-lipoxygenase upregulation by dexamethasone in human mast cells. *Biochem Biophys Res Commun* 265: 617–624

95 Funk CD, Hoshiko S, Matsumoto T, Rdmark O, Samuelsson B (1989) Characterization of the human 5-lipoxygenase gene. *Proc Natl Acad Sci USA* 86: 2587–2591

96 Hoshiko S, Radmark O, Samuelsson B (1990) Characterization of the human 5-lipoxygenase gene promoter. *Proc Natl Acad Sci USA* 87: 9073–9077

97 Boado RJ, Pardridge WM, Vinters HV, Black KL (1992) Differential expression of arachidonate 5-lipoxygenase transcripts in human brain tumors: Evidence for the expression of a multitranscript family. *Proc Natl Acad Sci USA* 89: 9044–9048

98 In KH, Asano K, Beier D, Grobholz J, Finn PW, Silverman EK, Silverman ES, Collins T, Fischer AR, Keith TP et al (1997) Naturally occurring mutations in the human 5-lipoxy-

genase gene promoter that modify transcription factor binding and reporter gene transcription. *J Clin Invest* 99: 1130–1137

99 Silverman ES, Du J, De Sanctis GT, Radmark O, Samuelsson B, Drazen JM, Collins T (1998) Egr-1 and sp1 interact functionally with the 5-lipoxygenase promoter and its naturally occurring mutants. *Am J Respir Cell Mol Biol* 19: 316–323

100 Drazen JM, Yandava CN, Dube L, Szczerback N, Hippensteel R, Pillari A, Israel E, Schork N, Silverman ES, Katz DA et al (1999) Pharmacogenetic association between alox5 promoter genotype and the response to anti-asthma treatment. *Nat Genet* 22: 168–170

101 Silverman E, In KH, Yandava C, Drazen JM (1998) Pharmacogenetics of the 5-lipoxygenase pathway in asthma. *Clin Exp Allergy* 28 (Suppl 5): 164–170; discussion 171–163

102 Drazen JM, Silverman ES (1999) Genetic determinants of 5-lipoxygenase transcription. *Int Arch Allergy Immunol* 118: 275–278

103 Silverman ES, Drazen JM (1999) The biology of 5-lipoxygenase: Function, structure, and regulatory mechanisms. *Proc Assoc Am Physicians* 111: 525–536

104 Silverman ES, Drazen JM (2000) Genetic variations in the 5-lipoxygenase core promoter. Description and functional implications. *Am J Respir Crit Care Med* 161: S77–80

105 Dixon RA, Diehl RE, Opas E, Rands E, Vickers PJ, Evans JF, Gillard JW, Miller DK (1990) Requirement of a 5-lipoxygenase-activating protein for leukotriene synthesis. *Nature* 343: 282–284

106 Kennedy B, Diehl R, Boie Y, Adam M, Dixon R (1991) Gene characterisation and promoter analysis of the human 5-lipoxygenase-activating protein (flap). *J Biol Chem* 266: 8511–8516

107 Yandava CN, Kennedy BP, Pillari A, Duncan AM, Drazen JM (1999) Cytogenetic and radiation hybrid mapping of human arachidonate 5-lipoxygenase-activating protein (alox5ap) to chromosome 13q12. *Genomics* 56: 131–133

108 Yoshida S, Penrose J, Stevenson D, Shikanani T, Asano K, Yandava C, Drazen J (2000) Polymorphism with genes in cysteinyl leukotriene synthesis pathway in aspirin-intolerant asthma. *Am J Respir Crit Care Med* 161 (3): A602 (abstract)

109 Lam BK, Penrose JF, Freeman GJ, Austen KF (1994) Expression cloning of a cdna for human leukotriene c4 synthase, an integral membrane protein conjugating reduced glutathione to leukotriene a4. *Proc Natl Acad Sci USA* 91: 7663–7667

110 Welsch DJ, Creely DP, Hauser SD, Mathis KJ, Krivi GG, Isakson PC (1994) Molecular cloning and expression of human leukotriene-c4 synthase. *Proc Natl Acad Sci USA* 91: 9745–9749

111 Scoggan KA, Jakobsson PJ, Ford-Hutchinson AW (1997) Production of leukotriene c4 in different human tissues is attributable to distinct membrane bound biosynthetic enzymes. *J Biol Chem* 272: 10182–10187

112 Bigby TD, Hodulik CR, Arden KC, Fu L (1996) Molecular cloning of the human leukotriene c4 synthase gene and assignment to chromosome 5q35. *Mol Med* 2: 637–646

113 Zhao JL, Austen KF, Lam BK (2000) Cell-specific transcription of leukotriene c(4) synthase involves a kruppel-like transcription factor and sp1. *J Biol Chem* 275: 8903–8910

114 Zaitsu M, Hamasaki Y, Yamamoto S, Kita M, Hayasaki R, Muro E, Kobayashi I, Matsuo M, Ichimaru T, Miyazaki S (1998) Effect of dexamethasone on leukotriene synthesis in dmso-stimulated hl-60 cells. *Prostaglandins Leukot Essent Fatty Acids* 59: 385–393

115 Riddick CA, Serio KJ, Hodulik CR, Ring WL, Regan MS, Bigby TD (1999) Tgf-beta increases leukotriene c4 synthase expression in the monocyte-like cell line, thp-1. *J Immunol* 162: 1101–1107

116 Shimada K, Navarro J, Goeger DE, Mustafa SB, Weigel PH, Weinman SA (1998) Expression and regulation of leukotriene-synthesis enzymes in rat liver cells. *Hepatology* 28: 1275–1281

117 Sanak M, Simon HU, Szczeklik A (1997) Leukotriene c4 synthase promoter polymorphism and risk of aspirin-induced asthma [letter]. *Lancet* 350: 1599–1600

118 Sanak M, Pierzchalska M, Bazan-Socha S, Szczeklik A (2000) Enhanced expression of the leukotriene c4 synthase due to overactive transcription of an allelic variant associated with aspirin-intolerant asthma. *Am J Respir Cell Mol Biol* 23: 290–296

119 Szczeklik A, Stevenson DD (1999) Aspirin-induced asthma: Advances in pathogenesis and management. *J Allergy Clin Immunol* 104: 5–13

120 Sampson A, Siddiqui S, Cowburn A, Buchanan D, Howarth P, Holgate S, Holloway J, Sayers I (2000) Variant ltc4 synthase allele modifies cysteinyl-leukotriene synthesis in eosinophils and predicts clinical response to zafarlukast. *Thorax* 55 (Suppl 2): S28–S31

121 Minami M, Ohno S, Kawasaki H, Radmark O, Samuelsson B, Jornvall H, Shimizu T, Seyama Y, Suzuki K (1987) Molecular cloning of a cdna coding for human leukotriene a4 hydrolase. Complete primary structure of an enzyme involved in eicosanoid synthesis. *J Biol Chem* 262: 13873–13876

122 Funk CD, Radmark O, Fu JY, Matsumoto T, Jornvall H, Shimizu T, Samuelsson B (1987) Molecular cloning and amino acid sequence of leukotriene a4 hydrolase. *Proc Natl Acad Sci USA* 84: 6677–6681

123 Mancini JA, Evans JF (1995) Cloning and characterization of the human leukotriene a4 hydrolase gene. *Eur J Biochem* 231: 65–71

124 Jendraschak E, Kaminski WE, Kiefl R, von Schacky C (1996) The human leukotriene a4 hydrolase gene is expressed in two alternatively spliced mrna forms. *Biochem J* 314: 733–737

125 Bulle F, Mattei MG, Siegrist S, Pawlak A, Passage E, Chobert MN, Laperche Y, Guellaen G (1987) Assignment of the human gamma-glutamyl transferase gene to the long arm of chromosome 22. *Hum Genet* 76: 283–286

126 Sakamuro D, Yamazoe M, Matsuda Y, Kangawa K, Taniguchi N, Matsuo H, Yoshikawa H, Ogasawara N (1988) The primary structure of human gamma-glutamyl transpeptidase. *Gene* 73: 1–9

127 Pawlak A, Wu SJ, Bulle F, Suzuki A, Chikhi N, Ferry N, Baik JH, Siegrist S, Guellaen G

(1989) Different gamma-glutamyl transpeptidase mrnas are expressed in human liver and kidney. *Biochem Biophys Res Commun* 164: 912–918

128 Kozak EM, Tate SS (1982) Glutathione-degrading enzymes of microvillus membranes. *J Biol Chem* 257: 6322–6327

129 Adachi H, Tawaragi Y, Inuzuka C, Kubota I, Tsujimoto M, Nishihara T, Nakazato H (1990) Primary structure of human microsomal dipeptidase deduced from molecular cloning. *J Biol Chem* 265: 3992–3995

130 Carter BZ, Wiseman AL, Orkiszewski R, Ballard KD, Ou CN, Lieberman MW (1997) Metabolism of leukotriene c4 in gamma-glutamyl transpeptidase-deficient mice. *J Biol Chem* 272: 12305–12310

131 Habib GM, Shi ZZ, Cuevas AA, Guo Q, Matzuk MM, Lieberman MW (1998) Leukotriene d4 and cystinyl-bis-glycine metabolism in membrane-bound dipeptidase-deficient mice. *Proc Natl Acad Sci USA* 95: 4859–4863

132 Owman C, Nilsson C, Lolait SJ (1996) Cloning of cdna encoding a putative chemoattractant receptor. *Genomics* 37: 187–194

133 Akbar GKM, Dasari VR, Webb TE, Ayyanathan K, Pillarisetti K, Sandhu AK, Athwal RS, Daniel JL, Ashby B, Barnard EA et al (1996) Molecular cloning of a novel p2 purinoceptor from human erythroleukemia cells. *J Biol Chem* 271: 18363–18367

134 Yokomizo T, Izumi T, Chang K, Takuwa Y, Shimizu T (1997) A g-protein-coupled receptor for leukotriene b4 that mediates chemotaxis. *Nature* 387: 620–624

135 Yokomizo T, Masuda K, Kato K, Toda A, Izumi T, Shimizu T (2000) Leukotriene b4 receptor. Cloning and intracellular signaling. *Am J Respir Crit Care Med* 161: S51-55

136 Pulleyn L, Adcock I, Barnes P (2000) A screen of the cyslt1 receptor gene for polymorphisms associated with asthma severity. American Thoracic Society, Toronto, meeting abstract

137 Bolk S, Lilly C, Yandava C, Green M, Lander E, Daly M, Evans J, Metzker M, Drazen J (2000) Naturally occuring sequence variants in the cyslt1 receptor. American Thoracic Society, Toronto, meeting abstract

138 Panettieri RA, Tan EM, Ciocca V, Luttmann MA, Leonard TB, Hay DW (1998) Effects of ltd4 on human airway smooth muscle cell proliferation, matrix expression, and contraction *in vitro*: Differential sensitivity to cysteinyl leukotriene receptor antagonists. *Am J Respir Cell Mol Biol* 19: 453–461

139 Malmstrom K, Rodriguez-Gomez G, Guerra J, Villaran C, Pineiro A, Wei LX, Seidenberg BC, Reiss TF (1999) Oral montelukast, inhaled beclomethasone, and placebo for chronic asthma. A randomized, controlled trial. Montelukast/beclomethasone study group. *Ann Intern Med* 130: 487–495

140 Hasday JD, Meltzer SS, Moore WC, Wisniewski P, Hebel JR, Lanni C, Dube LM, Bleecker ER (2000) Anti-inflammatory effects of zileuton in a subpopulation of allergic asthmatics. *Am J Respir Crit Care Med* 161: 1229–1236

141 Goulet JL, Byrum RS, Key ML, Nguyen M, Wagoner VA, Koller BH (2000) Genetic factors determine the contribution of leukotrienes to acute inflammatory responses. *J Immunol* 164: 4899–4907

Genetics of asthma severity

Ladina Joos, Peter D. Paré and Andrew J. Sandford

McDonald Research Laboratories/iCAPTURE Centre, University of British Columbia, St. Paul's Hospital, 1081 Burrard Street, Vancouver, B.C., Canada V6Z 1Y6

Introduction

There is strong evidence for a major hereditary contribution to the etiology of asthma and allergic diseases. However, only a few epidemiological studies have specifically addressed the genetic contribution to asthma severity. Sarafino et al. studied 39 monozygotic twin pairs and 55 same-sex dizygotic twin pairs who were between 2 and 20 years of age and had asthma present in at least one member of each pair [1]. In the 23 monozygotic and 13 dizygotic twins who were concordant for asthma, there was a significant correlation of asthma severity, defined as the product of attack frequency and an intensity rating, for monozygotic pairs but not for dizygotic pairs. This difference between monozygotic and dizygotic severity correlation was significant. Wilson et al. studied factors relating to the severity of symptoms at 5 years of age in 51 children with a history of severe wheeze in early childhood [2]. A positive family history of asthma was the only significant predictor of overall severity, defined by severity of attacks and interval symptom score, suggesting a genetic predisposition.

Asthma is a heterogeneous disease. Socioeconomic status, availability of medical treatment, concomitant diseases, the patient's compliance, and exposure to triggers such as allergens, cigarette smoke, or air pollution play a major role in modifying disease severity and control. Asthma severity has to be properly assessed, and severe asthma has to be distinguished from poorly controlled asthma if a genetic contribution to severity is to be discerned.

Assessing asthma severity

There is no gold standard in the assessment of asthma severity, partially because of confusion in the literature between the underlying biologic severity of disease and the current level of control. Severity can be separated into two components,

The Hereditary Basis of Allergic Diseases, edited by Stephen T. Holgate and John W. Holloway
© 2002 Birkhäuser Verlag Basel/Switzerland

one related to the frequency and intensity of asthma exacerbations and the other related to the chronicity and persistence of symptoms and functional abnormalities.

Aas was the first author to suggest a classification of asthmatics into subgroups, using frequency and severity of symptoms and lung function between attacks as parameters [3]. Currently, the most widely used guideline for quantifying severity in North America is the National Asthma Education and Prevention Program (NAEPP) Expert Panel II Guideline [4]. This score takes only four variables into account (Tab. 1) and is therefore easy to use. However, severity is assessed prior to treatment, and therefore asthmatics are categorized when they are poorly controlled. For this and other reasons, the NAEPP Guideline has been criticized repeatedly [5–7].

Other scores have been suggested to assess asthma severity. Redier et al. developed a computer-based Expert System that includes numerous variables, such as medical history, triggers, objective parameters, and current treatment [8]. Even though the authors showed a good correlation of their Expert System with disease severity assessed by specialists, this scoring system is cumbersome, requires specific equipment, and is not suitable for clinical practice.

Ideally, asthma severity should be defined by the minimum medication required to achieve adequate control rather than by symptoms and abnormal lung function, as suggested by Cockroft [7]. To date, there is no widely used algorithm that allows assessment of asthma severity according to these criteria. Only scores that incorporate the intensity of therapy as well as symptoms and lung function can hope to separate severity from lack of asthma control. Adequate therapy in severely affected patients can render them less symptomatic and functionally better than poorly controlled patients who have mild disease. Table 1 summarizes the different variables used in clinical scoring systems.

Candidate genes for asthma severity

The concept that there could be separate genetic control of the presence *versus* the severity of hereditary diseases is not new [9], and it is supported by the observation of marked phenotypic heterogeneity between individuals who have simple Mendelian disorders caused by the same mutant alleles [10, 11]. In complex genetic diseases such as asthma it may be difficult to distinguish causative genes from modifier genes, since it is likely that multiple genes are responsible for the phenotype and that environmental factors interact strongly with these susceptibility genes to modify the phenotype. One way to model the genetics of complex diseases is to assume that there is a normal distribution of liability to the disease in the population. The diagnosis of a disease occurs when a threshold of disease liability is reached. Disease severity may be the result of the total number of genetic risk fac-

Table 1 - Comparison of different clinical scores and their parameters

	NAEPP [4]	Expert system [8]	Aas [3]	Hargreave [41]	Cockroft [7]
FEV_1	+	+	−	+	−
PEF variability	+	+	−	+	−
Night symptoms	+	+	−	−	+
Daytime symptoms	+	+	+	+	+
β_2-agonist use	−	+	−	+	+
Inhaled corticosteroids	−	+	+	−	+
Systemic steroids in previous year	−	+	+	−	+
Dyspnea	−	+	+	+	−
Asthma control	−	−	−	−	+
Number of classes	4	5	5	4	5

PEF, peak expiratory flow

tors present within an individual and their interaction with each other and with the environment. Thus, it may be artificial to discuss candidate genes for severity separately from those suspected to cause asthma. However, for the purposes of this chapter, we have concentrated on studies in which the severity of asthma has been used as a phenotype.

Interleukin-4 and its receptor

Chromosome 5q contains numerous candidate genes that may play a role in airway inflammation associated with asthma. In particular, interleukin-4 (IL-4) is an attractive candidate gene on the basis of its involvement in IgE production and induction of inflammation. Several investigators have published data showing linkage of markers on chromosome 5q with the phenotypes of bronchial hyperresponsiveness [12] and/or total IgE levels [13].

IL-4 is secreted by Th2 lymphocytes and mast cells and is the major cytokine responsible for the induction of IgE synthesis by B cells [14]. In addition, it promotes the transformation of Th0 cells into the Th2 phenotype [15], leading to the secretion of more IL-4 and other Th2-derived cytokines, perpetuating the allergic cascade.

Two independent groups of investigators have addressed the involvement of the IL-4 gene in asthma severity. Burchard et al. investigated a C-589T polymorphism in the IL-4 promoter in 772 Caucasian and African American patients with asthma of varying severity [16]. There was a significantly different prevalence of the TT genotype in African Americans and Caucasians. Furthermore, in the Caucasians, there was a significant association of the mutant IL-4-589 T allele with an FEV_1 below 50% of predicted (odds ratio 1.4). The reason for this association remains to be determined since the T allele was not associated with increased total IgE levels. It is unclear why the authors chose a cut off of 50% predicted to categorize the asthma severity. Overall, this polymorphism accounts for only 0.6% of the variance of FEV_1 in the studied population. Furthermore, the patients enrolled in this study were selected to have an FEV_1 between 40% and 80% predicted and therefore represent only moderate and severe asthmatics.

Further evidence for the involvement of the IL-4 gene in asthma severity was found in a case-control study of 145 patients with allergic asthma and 160 healthy controls from Tunisia [17]. Patients were stratified into two groups: mild asthma and moderate/severe asthma, according to the NAEPP guideline [4], using FEV_1 and daytime and nighttime symptoms as variables. Genotype analysis for a three-allele repeat polymorphism in intron 2 of the IL-4 gene showed an increase of the A1/A3 genotype in asthmatics *versus* controls and a decrease of the A3/A3 genotype in the asthmatic group. Furthermore, the A1/A3 genotype was significantly more prevalent in the moderate/severe group when compared with the mild asthmatics (relative risk [RR] = 3.9), whereas the A3/A3 genotype was less frequent in moderate/severe asthmatics (RR = 0.2). There are no data to show a functional effect of this polymorphism on IL-4 gene expression. Most likely, this polymorphism is in linkage disequilibrium with another polymorphism in the IL-4 gene or in other genes on chromosome 5q. The genotype frequencies of these polymorphisms in ethnic groups other than Tunisian remain to be determined.

A polymorphism within the α-chain of the IL-4 receptor has been associated with atopy [18]. The same investigators who described this association genotyped 159 asthmatic individuals and 42 non-allergic control subjects to evaluate the influence of this polymorphism on asthma severity [19]. Asthma-severity categorization was performed according to the NAEPP guideline [4], but FEV_1 was used as the only variable. In the severe group ($FEV_1 < 60\%$ predicted), homozygosity for the mutant R576 allele was significantly more prevalent than in the mild group ($FEV_1 > 80\%$ predicted), and the mean FEV_1 was significantly lower in R576-homozygotes. These data suggest an involvement of this polymorphism in asthma severity; however, the molecular mechanism underlying the association remains to be determined.

β$_2$-adrenergic receptor

The involvement of the β$_2$-adrenergic receptor in bronchial asthma has been a long-standing hypothesis. Reihsaus and colleagues conducted a study to determine whether any variants of the gene could be detected and whether any of them were associated with asthma [20]. They found nine different point mutations, four of which caused amino-acid substitutions. None of these mutations was more prevalent in asthma patients than in normal control subjects. However, in the asthma group, one mutation (substitution of glycine for arginine at position 16) was correlated with more severe asthma, as indicated by the use of corticosteroids and immunization therapy. Green and associates performed *in vitro* studies to determine the functional significance of the different mutations [21]. The Gly16 mutant receptor significantly increased the degree of agonist-promoted downregulation of receptor expression. These data provide a reasonable explanation for the observed association with severe asthma because receptor downregulation could lead to an increased need for bronchodilators and inhaled steroids to control symptoms, suggesting more severe disease. This mutation has also been associated with nocturnal asthma [22]. Another polymorphism, resulting in a glutamine-to-glutamic-acid alteration at amino acid 27 (Gln27/Glu27), has been shown to render the receptor more resistant to agonist-induced downregulation [21]. This variant has been associated with less marked airway hyperresponsiveness in asthmatics [23, 24].

Weir and associates specifically addressed whether the Gln27 and Gly16 alleles predisposed to more severe asthma [25]. Patients were stratified into three different groups: mild and moderate, divided arbitrarily according to FEV_1 and steroid use, and fatal/near-fatal asthma, characterized by an attack leading to death or requiring intubation, respectively. The Gly16, Gln27, and Gly16/Gln27 haplotype were not more prevalent in fatal/near-fatal asthma compared with mild/moderate asthmatics. However, there was an increased prevalence of the Gln27 allele and the Gly16/Gln27 haplotype in the moderate asthmatics compared with the mild asthmatics. The lack of association with fatal/near-fatal asthma raises the question of the usefulness of this designation as a marker of severity. Although it is logical to assume that individuals with severe disease will be at risk of fatal or near-fatal episodes, it is also possible that these episodes are more indicative of poorly controlled asthma that is due to inappropriate management and/or poor patient compliance with therapy.

α_1-antitrypsin deficiency

Since the discovery of the strong association of α_1-antitrypsin (AAT) deficiency and pulmonary emphysema [26], a number of investigators have studied the involvement of AAT deficiency in asthma. There are two common alleles associated with AAT deficiency, denoted Z and S. Several groups have described increased prevalence of Z heterozygosity in asthmatics irrespective of severity [27, 28], while other studies have found no association between AAT variants and asthma [29, 30]. Katz et al. screened 151 children with severe asthma and 230 age-matched controls for

AAT deficiency and found a similar prevalence in both groups [31]. There was a greater proportion of Z heterozygotes in a subgroup of children with steroid-dependent asthma. However, this difference was not statistically significant. In a similar study, Lindmark et al. found a higher number of hospital admissions in asthmatic children heterozygous for the Z phenotype, but there was no increase in prevalence of this phenotype when compared with healthy children [32]. In another study, children who were heterozygous for the Z allele required more bronchodilators and long-term corticosteroid therapy [33].

Other candidate genes

TNFα is a potent proinflammatory cytokine expressed by a variety of cells in the airways. A TNFα promoter polymorphism, consisting of a G to A transition at position −308, has been shown to be associated with increased secretion of TNFα from macrophages *in vitro* [34]. Allele 2 of the polymorphism shows a higher prevalence in asthmatics compared with controls [35]. Chagani et al. found a higher prevalence of the polymorphism in moderate asthmatics compared with mild asthmatics and healthy controls. However, there was no increased prevalence in the group of fatal/near-fatal asthmatics compared with mild/moderate asthmatics [36]. In this study, the same patient data were used as in Weir et al. [25]; therefore, the same limitations apply.

Platelet-activating factor (PAF) has been implicated in the pathophysiology of inflammation in asthma because of its ability to activate inflammatory cells [37]. A deficiency in PAF acetylhydrolase, a PAF-degrading enzyme, has been associated with severe asthma, classified by the amount of respiratory symptoms, in Japanese children [38], Stafforini et al. found a point mutation near the active site of PAF acetylhydrolase that leads to the replacement of valine with phenylalanine at position 279, and this mutation results in an inactive enzyme [39]. The same group studied the prevalence of this mutation in 264 asthmatics and 263 healthy subjects from eastern Japan [40]. They found a higher prevalence of the Phe279 allele within the asthmatic group when compared with the healthy controls. Furthermore, Phe279 homozygotes were the genotypic group with largest proportion of severe asthmatics. However, the authors do not state whether these differences are statistically significant; therefore, the results, even though biologically plausible, must be interpreted with caution.

In summary, there is very limited evidence that there is a genetic contribution to asthma severity, largely because the question has not been systematically investigated. Because asthma, like other complex genetic diseases, is polygenic and because there is likely to be considerable genetic heterogeneity, it is logical to predict that different combinations of susceptibility genes would lead to phenotypic heterogeneity, including heterogeneity in severity. However, environmental factors including exposure to allergens and infections also contribute significantly to severity, and these environmental factors could overwhelm the influence of genes. What is needed to address this question are additional studies of the familial concordance and segregation of markers of asthma severity, correcting, if possible, for environmental modifiers. In the meantime, it is reasonable to examine the influence on severity of susceptibility genes for asthma using case-control studies. The ultimate hope is that specific gene variants will be found that predict an individual patient's risk for severe disease and thus aid in the clinical management of the patients.

Acknowledgements

Ladina Joos was supported by the Swiss National Science Foundation, the Novartis Research Foundation, the Uarda-Frutiger Foundation and the Swiss Society of Pneumology, and Andrew J. Sandford was supported by a Parker B. Francis Fellowship.

References

1   Sarafino EP, Goldfedder J (1995) Genetic factors in the presence, severity, and triggers of asthma. *Arch Dis Child* 73: 112–116

2   Wilson NM, Dore CJ, Silverman M (1997) Factors relating to the severity of symptoms at 5 yrs in children with severe wheeze in the first 2 yrs of life. *Eur Respir J* 10: 346–353

3   Aas K (1981) Heterogeneity of bronchial asthma. Sub-populations – or different stages of the disease. *Allergy* 36: 3–14

4   Expert Panel Report II (1997) Guidelines for the diagnosis and management of asthma. National Asthma Education and Prevention Program, National Institutes of Health, Bethesda, MD, NIH publication: 97-4051

5   Osborne ML, Vollmer WM, Pedula KL, Wilkins J, Buist AS, M OH (1999) Lack of correlation of symptoms with specialist-assessed long-term asthma severity. *Chest* 115: 85–91

6   Colice GL, Vanden Burgt J, Song J, Stampone P, Thompson PJ (1999) Categorizing asthma severity. *Am J Resp Crit Care Med* 160: 1962–1967

7   Cockcroft DW, Swystun VA (1996) Asthma control *versus* asthma severity. *J Allergy Clin Immunol* 98: 1016–1018

8   Redier H, Daures JP, Michel C, Proudhon H, Vervloet D, Charpin D, Marsac J, Dusser D, Brambilla C, Wallaert B et al (1995) Assessment of the severity of asthma by an expert system. Description and evaluation. *Am J Respir Crit Care Med* 151: 345–352

9   Romeo G, McKusick VA (1994) Phenotypic diversity, allelic series and modifier genes [news]. *Nat Genet* 7: 451–453

10 Rosenstein BJ (1994) Genotype-phenotype correlations in cystic fibrosis. *Lancet* 343: 746–747

11 Liechti-Gallati S, Bonsall I, Malik N, Schneider V, Kraemer LG, Ruedeberg A, Moser H, Kraemer R (1992) Genotype/phenotype association in cystic fibrosis: analyses of the delta F508, R553X, and 3905insT mutations. *Pediatr Res* 32: 175–178

12 Postma DS, Bleecker ER, Amelung PJ, Holroyd KJ, Xu J, Panhuysen CI, Meyers DA, Levitt RC (1995) Genetic susceptibility to asthma – bronchial hyperresponsiveness coinherited with a major gene for atopy. *N Engl J Med* 333: 894–900

13 Marsh DG, Neely JD, Breazeale DR, Ghosh B, Freidhoff LR, Ehrlich-Kautzky E, Schou C, Krishnaswamy G, Beaty TH (1994) Linkage analysis of IL4 and other chromosome 5q31.1 markers and total serum immunoglobulin E concentrations. *Science* 264: 1152–1156

14 Bonnefoy JY, Gauchat JF, Lecoanet-Henchoz S, Graber P, Aubry JP (1996) Regulation of human IgE synthesis. *Ann NY Acad Sci* 796: 59–71

15 Kopf M, Le Gros G, Bachmann M, Lamers MC, Bluethmann H, Kohler G (1993) Disruption of the murine IL-4 gene blocks Th2 cytokine responses. *Nature* 362: 245–248

16 Burchard EG, Silverman EK, Rosenwasser LJ, Borish L, Yandava C, Pillari A, Weiss ST, Hasday J, Lilly CM, Ford JG et al (1999) Association between a sequence variant in the IL-4 gene promoter and FEV(1) in asthma. *Am J Respir Crit Care Med* 160: 919–922

17 Chouchane L, Sfar I, Bousaffara R, El Kamel A, Sfar MT, Ismail A (1999) A repeat polymorphism in interleukin-4 gene is highly associated with specific clinical phenotypes of asthma. *Int Arch Allergy Immunol* 120: 50–55

18 Hershey GK, Friedrich MF, Esswein LA, Thomas ML, Chatila TA (1997) The association of atopy with a gain-of-function mutation in the alpha subunit of the interleukin-4 receptor. *N Engl J Med* 337: 1720–1725

19 Rosa-Rosa L, Zimmermann N, Bernstein JA, Rothenberg ME, Hershey GKK (1999) The R576 IL-4 receptor alpha allele correlates with asthma severity. *J Allergy Clin Immunol* 104: 1008–1014

20 Reihsaus E, Innis M, MacIntyre N, Liggett SB (1993) Mutations in the gene encoding for the β_2-adrenergic receptor in normal and asthmatic subjects. *Am J Respir Cell Mol Biol* 8: 334–339

21 Green SA, Turki J, Bejarano P, Hall IP, Liggett SB (1995) Influence of β_2-adrenergic receptor genotypes on signal transduction in human airway smooth muscle cells. *Am J Respir Cell Mol Biol* 13: 25–33

22 Turki J, Pak J, Green SA, Martin RJ, Liggett SB (1995) Genetic polymorphisms of the β_2-adrenergic receptor in nocturnal and nonnocturnal asthma. Evidence that Gly16 correlates with the nocturnal phenotype. *J Clin Invest* 95: 1635–1641

23 Hall IP, Wheatley A, Wilding P, Liggett SB (1995) Association of Glu 27 β_2-adrenoceptor polymorphism with lower airway reactivity in asthmatic subjects. *Lancet* 345: 1213–1214

24 Ramsay CE, Hayden CM, Tiller KJ, Burton PR, Goldblatt J, Lesouef PN (1999) Polymorphisms in the beta2-adrenoreceptor gene are associated with decreased airway responsiveness. *Clin Exp Allergy* 29: 1195–1203

25 Weir TD, Mallek N, Sandford AJ, Bai TR, Awadh N, FitzGerald JM, Cockcroft D,

James A, Liggett SB, Paré PD (1998) β$_2$-adrenergic receptor haplotypes in mild, moderate and fatal/near fatal asthma. *Am J Respir Crit Care Med* 158: 787–791

26 Laurell CC, Eriksson S (1963) The electrophorectic α$_1$-globulin pattern of serum in α$_1$-antitrypsin deficiency. *Scand J Clin Lab Invest* 15: 132–140

27 Buist AS, Sexton GJ, Azzam AM, Adams BE (1979) Pulmonary function in heterozygotes for α$_1$-antitrypsin deficiency: a case-control study. *Am Rev Respir Dis* 120: 759–766

28 Hoffmann JJ, Kramps JA, Dijkman JH (1981) Intermediate α$_1$-antitrypsin deficiency in atopic allergy. *Clin Allergy* 11: 555–560

29 Welch MH, Reinecke ME, Hammarsten JF, Guenter CA (1969) Antitrypsin deficiency in pulmonary disease: the significance of intermediate levels. *Ann Intern Med* 71: 533–542

30 Webb DR, Hyde RW, Schwartz RH, Hall WJ, Condemi JJ, Townes PL (1973) Serum α$_1$-antitrypsin variants. Prevalence and clinical spirometry. *Am Rev Respir Dis* 108: 918–925

31 Katz RM, Lieberman J, Siegel SC (1976) α$_1$ antitrypsin levels and prevalence of Pi variant phenotypes in asthmatic children. *J Allergy Clin Immunol* 57: 41–45

32 Lindmark B, Svenonius E, Eriksson S (1990) Heterozygous α$_1$-antichymotrypsin and PiZ α$_1$-antitrypsin deficiency. Prevalence and clinical spectrum in asthmatic children. *Allergy* 45: 197–203

33 Hyde JS, Werner P, Kumar CM, Moore BS (1979) Protease inhibitor variants in children and young adults with chronic asthma. *Ann Allergy* 43: 8–13

34 Wilson AG, Symons JA, McDowell TL, McDevitt HO, Duff GW (1997) Effects of a polymorphism in the human tumor necrosis factor a promoter on transcriptional activation. *Proc Natl Acad Sci USA* 94: 3195–3199

35 Moffatt MF, Cookson WOCM (1997) Tumour necrosis factor haplotypes and asthma. *Hum Mol Genet* 6: 551–554

36 Chagani T, Pare PD, Zhu S, Weir TD, Bai TR, Behbehani NA, Fitzgerald JM, Sandford AJ (1999) Prevalence of tumor necrosis factor-alpha and angiotensin converting enzyme polymorphisms in mild/moderate and fatal/near-fatal asthma. *Am J Respir Crit Care Med* 160: 278–282

37 Page CP (1988) The role of platelet-activating factor in asthma. *J Allergy Clin Immunol* 81: 144–152

38 Miwa M, Miyake T, Yamanaka T, Sugatani J, Suzuki Y, Sakata S, Araki Y, Matsumoto M (1988) Characterization of serum platelet-activating factor (PAF) acetylhydrolase. Correlation between deficiency of serum PAF acetylhydrolase and respiratory symptoms in asthmatic children. *J Clin Invest* 82: 1983–1991

39 Stafforini DM, Satoh K, Atkinson DL, Tjoelker LW, Eberhardt C, Yoshida H, Imaizumi T, Takamatsu S, Zimmerman GA, McIntyre TM et al (1996) Platelet-activating factor acetylhydrolase deficiency. A missense mutation near the active site of an anti-inflammatory phospholipase. *J Clin Invest* 97: 2784–2791

40 Stafforini DM, Numao T, Tsodikov A, Vaitkus D, Fukuda T, Watanabe N, Fueki N,

McIntyre TM, Zimmerman GA, Makino S et al (1999) Deficiency of platelet-activating factor acetylhydrolase is a severity factor for asthma. *J Clin Invest* 103: 989–997

41   Hargreave FE, Dolovich J, Newhouse MT (1990) The assessment and treatment of asthma: a conference report. *J Allergy Clin Immunol* 85: 1098–1111

Index

The PIR-Series
Progress in Inflammation Research

Homepage: http://www.birkhauser.ch

Up-to-date information on the latest developments in the pathology, mechanisms and therapy of inflammatory disease are provided in this monograph series. Areas covered include vascular responses, skin inflammation, pain, neuroinflammation, arthritis cartilage and bone, airways inflammation and asthma, allergy, cytokines and inflammatory mediators, cell signalling, and recent advances in drug therapy. Each volume is edited by acknowledged experts providing succinct overviews on specific topics intended to inform and explain. The series is of interest to academic and industrial biomedical researchers, drug development personnel and rheumatologists, allergists, pathologists, dermatologists and other clinicians requiring regular scientific updates.

Available volumes:

T Cells in Arthritis, P. Miossec, W. van den Berg, G. Firestein (Editors), 1998
Chemokines and Skin, E. Kownatzki, J. Norgauer (Editors), 1998
Medicinal Fatty Acids, J. Kremer (Editor), 1998
Inducible Enzymes in the Inflammatory Response, D.A. Willoughby, A. Tomlinson (Editors), 1999
Cytokines in Severe Sepsis and Septic Shock, H. Redl, G. Schlag (Editors), 1999
Fatty Acids and Inflammatory Skin Diseases, J.-M. Schröder (Editor), 1999
Immunomodulatory Agents from Plants, H. Wagner (Editor), 1999
Cytokines and Pain, L. Watkins, S. Maier (Editors), 1999
In Vivo *Models of Inflammation*, D. Morgan, L. Marshall (Editors), 1999
Pain and Neurogenic Inflammation, S.D. Brain, P. Moore (Editors), 1999
Anti-Inflammatory Drugs in Asthma, A.P. Sampson, M.K. Church (Editors), 1999
Novel Inhibitors of Leukotrienes, G. Folco, B. Samuelsson, R.C. Murphy (Editors), 1999
Vascular Adhesion Molecules and Inflammation, J.D. Pearson (Editor), 1999
Metalloproteinases as Targets for Anti-Inflammatory Drugs, K.M.K. Bottomley, D. Bradshaw, J.S. Nixon (Editors), 1999
Free Radicals and Inflammation, P.G. Winyard, D.R. Blake, C.H. Evans (Editors), 1999
Gene Therapy in Inflammatory Diseases, C.H. Evans, P. Robbins (Editors), 2000
New Cytokines as Potential Drugs, S. K. Narula, R. Coffmann (Editors), 2000
High Throughput Screening for Novel Anti-inflammatories, M. Kahn (Editor), 2000
Immunology and Drug Therapy of Atopic Skin Diseases, C.A.F. Bruijnzeel-Komen, E.F. Knol (Editors), 2000
Novel Cytokine Inhibitors, G.A. Higgs, B. Henderson (Editors), 2000
Inflammatory Processes. Molecular Mechanisms and Therapeutic Opportunities, L.G. Letts, D.W. Morgan (Editors), 2000

Cellular Mechanisms in Airways Inflammation, C. Page, K. Banner, D. Spina (Editors), 2000
Inflammatory and Infectious Basis of Atherosclerosis, J.L. Mehta (Editor), 2001
Muscarinic Receptors in Airways Diseases, J. Zaagsma, H. Meurs, A.F. Roffel (Editors), 2001
TGF-β and Related Cytokines in Inflammation, S.N. Breit, S. Wahl (Editors), 2001
Nitric Oxide and Inflammation, D. Salvemini, T.R. Billiar, Y. Vodovotz (Editors), 2001
Neuroinflammatory Mechanisms in Alzheimer's Disease. Basic and Clinical Research, J. Rogers (Editor), 2001
Disease-modifying Therapy in Vasculitides, C.G.M. Kallenberg, J.W. Cohen Tervaert (Editors), 2001
Inflammation and Stroke, G.Z. Feuerstein (Editor), 2001
NMDA Antagonists as Potential Analgesic Drugs, D.J.S. Sirinathsinghji, R.G. Hill (Editors), 2002
Migraine: A Neuroinflammatory Disease? E.L.H. Spierings, M. Sanchez del Rio (Editors), 2002
Mechanisms and Mediators of Neuropathic Pain, A.B. Malmberg, S.R. Chaplan (Editors), 2002
Bone Morphogenetic Proteins: From Laboratory to Clinical Practice, S. Vukicevic, K.T. Sampath (Editors), 2002